OSTEOPOROSIS DIET COOKBOOK

for Seniors

2024

SAY BYE TO
BONE PAIN,
LOSS OF HEIGHT,
STOOPED POSTURE,
FRACTURES, REDUCED GRIP STRENGTH,
RECEDING GUMS AND TOOTH LOSS

28- DAY MEAL PLAN INCLUDED

BY JUDY KELLY

Strong Bones After 60

Osteoporosis Diet Cookbook for Seniors

Nutrient-Packed Recipes, Whole Foods to Relieve Joint Pain, Boost Bone Health and Density, Enhance Mobility, Reduce Fracture Risks, and Enjoy a Flavorful Aging. Plus, a 28-Day Meal Plan to Reverse Osteoporosis.

Judy Kelly

Table of Contents

Introduction

- **Welcome to Bone-Healthy Cooking**

Hello Dear Readers,

Step into the world of delicious and nutritious meals designed just for you—welcome to Bone-Healthy Cooking! This cookbook is all about celebrating good food that not only tastes great but also takes care of your bones, keeping them strong and healthy.

Now, we know food is more than just fuel; it's like a secret potion that helps keep our bones in top shape. Each recipe here is made with ingredients that your bones will love, and we've kept things simple and enjoyable because good health should be a joy, not a chore.

Whether you're a kitchen pro or just getting started, don't worry—this cookbook is like having a friendly guide by your side. From breakfast to dinner, we've got recipes that bring together flavors and nutrition, all with your bone health in mind.

But this cookbook is more than just about what happens in the kitchen. It's an invitation to think about your health in a whole new way. As you try out these tasty recipes, remember that every bite is a small but important step toward keeping your bones strong and happy.

Thanks a bunch for letting us be part of your kitchen adventures. We hope this cookbook brings you inspiration, tasty meals, and a little extra joy in every bite.

Here's to your health, happiness, and the joy of Bone-Healthy Cooking!

Warm regards,

Judy Kelly.

How to Use This Cookbook

Navigating a cookbook can be as enjoyable as cooking itself! Here's a simple guide to help you make the most out of Bone-Healthy Cooking and turn every meal into a delightful, bone-nourishing experience.

1. Take a Friendly Stroll:

Start by flipping through the pages. Get a feel for the recipes and notice the vibrant images that accompany them. This is your cookbook, and we want it to spark your excitement.

2. Mark Your Favorites:

As you browse, mark recipes that catch your eye. Maybe it's the picture of the creamy berry smoothie or the description of the comforting lentil soup. These will be your go-to recipes, so let's make them easy to find.

3. Check for Handy Tips:

Throughout the cookbook, you'll find handy tips and tricks. Look out for suggestions on ingredient substitutions, cooking techniques, or ways to personalize the recipes. These little nuggets of wisdom are here to make your cooking experience even more enjoyable.

4. Plan Your Meals:

Take a moment to plan your meals for the week. Maybe you want to start with the spinach and feta omelet for breakfast or the baked salmon with lemon and dill for dinner. Planning ahead can make your grocery shopping more efficient.

5. Make It Your Own:

Recipes are like guidelines, not strict rules. Feel free to add a little more of what you love or switch ingredients based on what's in your kitchen. Cooking is an art, and this cookbook is your canvas.

6. Gather What You Need:

Before you start cooking, gather all your ingredients and tools. Having everything in one place will make the process smoother, and you won't have to do a frantic search for that essential spice halfway through.

7. Enjoy the Process:

Cooking is not just about the final dish; it's about the journey. Take your time, enjoy the aromas, and savor the process. Cooking can be a therapeutic and fulfilling activity.

8. Share the Joy:

If you find a recipe you love, share it with friends or family. Maybe you can cook a meal together or surprise them with a tasty treat. Sharing good food is sharing joy.

9. Listen to Your Body:

Everyone's body is unique. Pay attention to how certain foods make you feel. If something doesn't work for you, feel free to make adjustments. This cookbook is here to support you in creating meals that suit your individual needs.

10. Connect with Us:

We'd love to hear about your cooking adventures! Connect with us through social media or our website. Share your favorite recipes, ask questions, or simply drop by to say hello. Your feedback is our inspiration.

This cookbook is more than just recipes; it's a companion on your journey to healthier, happier eating. May your kitchen be filled with laughter, delicious aromas, and the joy of creating meals that nourish your bones and your soul.

Happy Cooking!

Tips for Building Strong Bones through Nutrition

As we gracefully age, maintaining bone health becomes increasingly important. Strong bones contribute not only to physical well-being but also to an active and vibrant lifestyle. Here are some tips to support bone health through nutrition:

1. Embrace Calcium-Rich Foods:

Ensure your diet includes plenty of calcium-rich foods. Dairy products like milk, yogurt, and cheese are excellent sources. If you're lactose intolerant or prefer non-dairy options, explore fortified plant-based milk alternatives, leafy greens, and fish such as salmon and sardines.

2. Welcome the Sunshine Vitamin - Vitamin D:

Vitamin D plays a crucial role in calcium absorption. Embrace sunlight when possible, as your skin naturally produces vitamin D in response to sunlight exposure. Include vitamin D-rich foods like fatty fish (salmon, mackerel), egg yolks, and fortified foods in your diet. If needed, consult your healthcare provider about vitamin D supplements.

3. Prioritize Vitamin K:

Vitamin K is vital for bone health as it helps in bone mineralization. Include leafy green vegetables like kale, spinach, and Brussels sprouts in your meals to ensure an adequate intake of vitamin K.

4. Magnesium and Phosphorus Balance:

Magnesium and phosphorus work alongside calcium to support bone health. Incorporate nuts, seeds, whole grains, and lean meats into your diet for a balanced intake of these minerals.

5. Protein is Your Friend:

Adequate protein intake is essential for maintaining bone health. Include lean protein sources such as poultry, fish, beans, and tofu in your meals to support bone structure and strength.

6. Limit Sodium Intake:

High sodium consumption can lead to calcium loss from bones. Minimize processed and salty foods, and opt for fresh, whole foods seasoned with herbs and spices for flavor.

7. Moderate Caffeine and Alcohol:

While moderate caffeine and alcohol consumption is generally considered safe, excessive intake may interfere with calcium absorption. Keep these beverages in check and ensure they are part of a balanced diet.

8. Hydrate with Water:

Hydration is essential for overall health, including bone health. Water supports the proper functioning of cells involved in bone formation and remodeling. Aim for adequate daily water intake.

9. Omega-3 Fatty Acids for Inflammation Control:

Include omega-3 fatty acids in your diet, found in fatty fish (like salmon and mackerel), flaxseeds, and walnuts. These fatty acids have anti-inflammatory properties, which can contribute to overall bone health.

10. Maintain a Healthy Weight:

Achieving and maintaining a healthy weight is crucial for bone health. Being underweight can lead to bone loss, while excessive weight can strain bones. Aim for a balanced and sustainable weight for your body.

11. Stay Active:

Regular weight-bearing exercises, such as walking or strength training, contribute to bone density. Combine proper nutrition with physical activity for comprehensive bone health.

Remember, small changes in your diet can make a big difference over time. Consult with a healthcare professional or a nutritionist for personalized advice based on your specific needs and health conditions.

Chapter 1: Breakfast Boosters

1. Creamy Berry Smoothie Bowl

Ingredients:
- 1 cup mixed berries (strawberries, blueberries, raspberries)
- 1 banana, frozen
- 1/2 cup low-fat Greek yogurt
- 1/4 cup almond milk
- 1 tablespoon chia seeds
- 1 tablespoon honey
- 1/4 cup granola (for topping)

Instructions:
1. Blend the mixed berries, frozen banana, Greek yogurt, almond milk, and chia seeds until smooth.
2. Pour the smoothie into a bowl.
3. Drizzle honey over the top and sprinkle with granola.
4. Enjoy with a spoon!

---

2. Spinach and Feta Omelette

Ingredients:
- 2 eggs
- 1/4 cup fresh spinach, chopped
- 2 tablespoons feta cheese, crumbled
- 1 tablespoon olive oil
- Salt and pepper to taste

Instructions:
1. Whisk the eggs in a bowl and season with salt and pepper.
2. Heat olive oil in a pan over medium heat.
3. Pour the eggs into the pan and swirl to coat evenly.
4. Add chopped spinach and crumbled feta to one half of the omelette.
5. Fold the other half over the filling and cook until the eggs are set.
6. Slide the omelette onto a plate and serve.

---

3. Overnight Oats with Almonds and Dried Fruits

Ingredients:
- 1/2 cup rolled oats
- 1/2 cup almond milk
- 1 tablespoon chia seeds
- 2 tablespoons sliced almonds
- 2 tablespoons dried cranberries
- 1 teaspoon honey

Instructions:
1. Mix rolled oats, almond milk, and chia seeds in a jar.
2. Refrigerate overnight.
3. In the morning, stir in sliced almonds and dried cranberries.
4. Drizzle with honey before serving.

---

4. Greek Yogurt Parfait with Nuts and Berries

Ingredients:
- 1 cup Greek yogurt
- 1/2 cup mixed berries (strawberries, blueberries, raspberries)
- 2 tablespoons chopped nuts (almonds, walnuts)
- 1 tablespoon honey

Instructions:
1. Layer Greek yogurt in a glass or bowl.
2. Add a layer of mixed berries.
3. Sprinkle chopped nuts on top.
4. Repeat the layers.
5. Drizzle with honey before serving.

---

5. Quinoa and Chickpea Salad

Ingredients:
- 1/2 cup cooked quinoa
- 1/2 cup canned chickpeas, drained
- 1/4 cup cucumber, diced
- 1/4 cup cherry tomatoes, halved
- 2 tablespoons feta cheese, crumbled
- 1 tablespoon olive oil
- Fresh lemon juice, to taste
- Salt and pepper to taste

Instructions:
1. In a bowl, combine quinoa, chickpeas, cucumber, cherry tomatoes, and feta cheese.
2. Drizzle with olive oil and fresh lemon juice.
3. Season with salt and pepper.
4. Toss gently and enjoy.

---

6. Grilled Chicken Caesar Wrap

Ingredients:
- 1 whole-grain wrap
- 3 ounces grilled chicken breast, sliced
- 1 cup romaine lettuce, chopped
- 2 tablespoons Caesar dressing
- 1 tablespoon Parmesan cheese, grated

Instructions:
1. Lay the wrap flat and add sliced grilled chicken.
2. Top with chopped romaine lettuce.
3. Drizzle with Caesar dressing.
4. Sprinkle with grated Parmesan cheese.
5. Roll up the wrap and slice before serving.

---

7. Lentil Soup with Leafy Greens

Ingredients:
- 1 cup cooked lentils

- 1/2 cup spinach, chopped
- 1/4 cup kale, chopped
- 1 carrot, diced
- 1 celery stalk, diced
- 1 clove garlic, minced
- 4 cups vegetable broth
- Salt and pepper to taste

Instructions:
1. In a pot, sauté garlic, carrots, and celery until softened.
2. Add cooked lentils and vegetable broth.
3. Bring to a simmer and add chopped spinach and kale.
4. Season with salt and pepper.
5. Cook until the greens are wilted. Serve hot.

---

8. Tuna and Avocado Salad

Ingredients:
- 1 can tuna, drained
- 1 avocado, diced
- 1/4 cup red onion, finely chopped
- 1/4 cup cherry tomatoes, halved
- 2 tablespoons olive oil
- Fresh lemon juice, to taste
- Salt and pepper to taste

Instructions:
1. In a bowl, combine drained tuna, diced avocado, chopped red onion, and halved cherry tomatoes.

2. Drizzle with olive oil and fresh lemon juice.
3. Season with salt and pepper.
4. Toss gently and enjoy on whole-grain toast or crackers.

---

9. Baked Salmon with Lemon and Dill

Ingredients:
- 4 ounces salmon fillet
- 1 tablespoon olive oil
- 1 tablespoon fresh dill, chopped
- 1 lemon, sliced
- Salt and pepper to taste

Instructions:
1. Preheat the oven to 375°F (190°C).
2. Place the salmon fillet on a baking sheet.
3. Drizzle with olive oil and sprinkle with chopped dill.
4. Season with salt and pepper.
5. Arrange lemon slices on top of the salmon.
6. Bake for 15-20 minutes or until the salmon is cooked through.

---

10. Vegetarian Stir-Fry with Tofu and Broccoli

Ingredients:
- 1 cup firm tofu, cubed
- 1 cup broccoli florets
- 1/2 cup bell peppers, sliced

- 1/4 cup carrots, julienned
- 2 tablespoons soy sauce
- 1 tablespoon sesame oil
- 1 teaspoon ginger, minced
- 1 clove garlic, minced

Instructions:
1. In a wok or skillet, heat sesame oil over medium-high heat.
2. Add minced ginger and garlic, stir-fry for 30 seconds.
3. Add tofu cubes and cook until golden brown.
4. Add broccoli, bell peppers, and carrots. Stir-fry until vegetables are tender-crisp.
5. Pour in soy sauce and toss to combine.
6. Serve hot over brown rice or quinoa.

---

11. Whole Grain Pancakes with Berries

Ingredients:
- 1 cup whole wheat flour
- 1 tablespoon baking powder
- 1 tablespoon honey
- 1 cup almond milk
- 1 egg
- 1 cup mixed berries (blueberries, raspberries)

Instructions:
1. In a bowl, mix whole wheat flour and baking powder.
2. Add honey, almond milk, and egg. Stir until smooth.
3. Heat a griddle or pan and pour batter for each pancake.

4. Cook until bubbles form, then flip and cook until golden.
5. Serve with mixed berries on top.

---

12. Mushroom and Swiss Omelette

Ingredients:
- 2 eggs
- 1/4 cup mushrooms, sliced
- 2 tablespoons Swiss cheese, shredded
- 1 tablespoon olive oil
- Salt and pepper to taste

Instructions:
1. Whisk eggs and season with salt and pepper.
2. In a pan, sauté sliced mushrooms in olive oil until tender.
3. Pour whisked eggs over mushrooms.
4. Sprinkle shredded Swiss cheese on one side and fold the omelette.
5. Cook until eggs are set. Serve hot.

---

13. Fortified Orange Smoothie

Ingredients:
- 2 oranges, peeled and segmented
- 1/2 cup Greek yogurt
- 1 tablespoon honey
- 1/2 cup ice cubes

Instructions:
1. Blend orange segments, Greek yogurt, honey, and ice cubes until smooth.
2. Pour into a glass and enjoy this vitamin C-packed smoothie.

---

14. Golden Turmeric Latte

Ingredients:
- 1 cup almond milk
- 1 teaspoon turmeric powder
- 1/2 teaspoon cinnamon
- 1 teaspoon honey
- 1/2 teaspoon vanilla extract

Instructions:
1. Heat almond milk, turmeric, cinnamon, honey, and vanilla extract in a saucepan.
2. Whisk until frothy.
3. Pour into a mug and savor this warming turmeric latte.

---

15. Creamy Broccoli and Cheddar Soup

Ingredients:
- 1 cup broccoli florets
- 1/2 cup cheddar cheese, shredded
- 1 cup vegetable broth

- 1/2 cup milk
- 1 tablespoon butter
- Salt and pepper to taste

Instructions:
1. Steam broccoli until tender.
2. In a pot, melt butter and add steamed broccoli.
3. Pour in vegetable broth and milk. Simmer.
4. Blend until smooth and stir in cheddar cheese.
5. Season with salt and pepper. Serve hot.

---

16. Yogurt Parfait with Berries and Almonds

Ingredients:
- 1 cup plain yogurt
- 1/2 cup granola
- 1/2 cup mixed berries (strawberries, blueberries)
- 2 tablespoons sliced almonds

Instructions:
1. Layer plain yogurt in a glass or bowl.
2. Add a layer of granola and mixed berries.
3. Repeat the layers and top with sliced almonds.

---

17. Grilled Sardines with Citrus Marinade

Ingredients:

- 4 fresh sardine fillets
- 2 tablespoons olive oil
- 1 tablespoon orange juice
- 1 tablespoon lemon juice
- 1 teaspoon fresh thyme, chopped
- Salt and pepper to taste

Instructions:
1. In a bowl, mix olive oil, orange juice, lemon juice, and chopped thyme.
2. Season sardine fillets with salt and pepper.
3. Grill sardines, basting with the citrus marinade until cooked.

---

18. Mushroom and Swiss Omelette

Ingredients:
- 2 eggs
- 1/4 cup mushrooms, sliced
- 2 tablespoons Swiss cheese, shredded
- 1 tablespoon olive oil
- Salt and pepper to taste

Instructions:
1. Whisk eggs and season with salt and pepper.
2. In a pan, sauté sliced mushrooms in olive oil until tender.
3. Pour whisked eggs over mushrooms.
4. Sprinkle shredded Swiss cheese on one side and fold the omelette.
5. Cook until eggs are set. Serve hot.

---

19. Sun-Dried Tomato and Basil Quinoa Salad

Ingredients:
- 1 cup cooked quinoa
- 1/4 cup sun-dried tomatoes, chopped
- 1/4 cup fresh basil, chopped
- 2 tablespoons feta cheese, crumbled
- 1 tablespoon balsamic vinegar
- 1 tablespoon olive oil

Instructions:
1. In a bowl, combine cooked quinoa, sun-dried tomatoes, fresh basil, and crumbled feta.
2. Drizzle with balsamic vinegar and olive oil.
3. Toss gently and enjoy this flavorful quinoa salad.

---

20. Almond-Crusted Tilapia

Ingredients:
- 2 tilapia fillets
- 1/4 cup almond meal
- 1 tablespoon Dijon mustard
- 1 tablespoon olive oil
- 1 teaspoon lemon zest
- Salt and pepper to taste

Instructions:
1. Preheat the oven to 400°F (200°C).
2. In a bowl, mix almond meal, Dijon mustard, olive oil, lemon zest, salt, and pepper.
3. Coat tilapia fillets with the almond mixture.
4. Bake for 12-15 minutes or until fish flakes easily.

---

21. Decaf Green Tea Smoothie

Ingredients:
- 1 decaf green tea bag
- 1 cup almond milk
- 1/2 banana, frozen
- 1/2 cup pineapple chunks
- 1 tablespoon chia seeds
- Ice cubes

Instructions:
1. Brew the decaf green tea and let it cool.
2. In a blender, combine the cooled tea, almond milk, frozen banana, pineapple chunks, and chia seeds.
3. Blend until smooth, add ice cubes, and blend again.
4. Pour into a glass and enjoy this refreshing green tea smoothie.

—

22. Fresh Mint and Cucumber Infused Water

Ingredients:
- 1/2 cucumber, sliced
- 1/4 cup fresh mint leaves
- Ice cubes
- Water

Instructions:
1. In a pitcher, combine cucumber slices and fresh mint leaves.
2. Add ice cubes and fill the pitcher with water.
3. Allow it to infuse in the refrigerator for a few hours.
4. Serve chilled for a hydrating start to your day.

---

23. Vegetarian Breakfast Burrito

Ingredients:
- 1 whole-grain tortilla
- 1/2 cup black beans, cooked
- 1/4 cup diced tomatoes
- 2 tablespoons salsa
- 2 tablespoons shredded cheddar cheese
- 1 tablespoon cilantro, chopped

Instructions:
1. Warm the tortilla in a pan or microwave.
2. Layer with black beans, diced tomatoes, salsa, shredded cheddar cheese, and chopped cilantro.
3. Roll it up, and your hearty breakfast burrito is ready to enjoy.

---

24. Chia Seed Pudding with Mango

Ingredients:
- 2 tablespoons chia seeds
- 1/2 cup almond milk
- 1/2 teaspoon vanilla extract
- 1 tablespoon honey
- 1/2 cup fresh mango, diced

Instructions:
1. In a jar, mix chia seeds, almond milk, vanilla extract, and honey.
2. Refrigerate overnight.
3. In the morning, layer with diced mango for a delightful chia seed pudding.

---

25. Baked Avocado and Egg Cups

Ingredients:
- 2 avocados, halved and pitted
- 4 eggs
- Salt and pepper to taste
- Chopped chives for garnish

Instructions:
1. Preheat the oven to 375°F (190°C).

2. Scoop out some flesh from each avocado half to create a well.
3. Crack an egg into each avocado half.
4. Sprinkle with salt and pepper.
5. Bake for 12-15 minutes or until the eggs are set.
6. Garnish with chopped chives and serve.

---

26. Blueberry and Almond Baked Oatmeal Cups

Ingredients:
- 2 cups rolled oats
- 1/2 cup almond butter
- 1/4 cup honey
- 1 cup almond milk
- 1 teaspoon vanilla extract
- 1 cup blueberries

Instructions:
1. Preheat the oven to 350°F (175°C) and grease a muffin tin.
2. In a bowl, mix rolled oats, almond butter, honey, almond milk, and vanilla extract.
3. Gently fold in blueberries.
4. Spoon the mixture into the muffin tin and bake for 20-25 minutes.
5. Allow to cool before serving.

---

27. Cottage Cheese and Pineapple Skewers

Ingredients:
- 1 cup low-fat cottage cheese
- 1 cup pineapple chunks
- Wooden skewers

Instructions:
1. Thread alternating pieces of cottage cheese and pineapple onto wooden skewers.
2. Serve these tasty skewers for a protein-packed and fruity breakfast.

---

28. Mixed Nuts and Seeds Trail Mix

Ingredients:
- 1/2 cup almonds
- 1/4 cup walnuts
- 1/4 cup pumpkin seeds
- 1/4 cup dried cranberries
- 1/4 cup dark chocolate chips

Instructions:
1. Mix almonds, walnuts, pumpkin seeds, dried cranberries, and dark chocolate chips in a bowl.
2. Portion into small bags for a convenient and nutritious on-the-go breakfast.

---

29. Baked Apple with Cinnamon and Walnuts

Ingredients:
- 2 apples, cored and halved
- 1 teaspoon cinnamon
- 2 tablespoons chopped walnuts
- 1 tablespoon honey

Instructions:
1. Preheat the oven to 375°F (190°C).
2. Place apple halves in a baking dish.
3. Sprinkle with cinnamon and top with chopped walnuts.
4. Drizzle with honey.
5. Bake for 20-25 minutes or until apples are tender.

---

30. Dark Chocolate-Dipped Strawberries

Ingredients:
- 1 cup fresh strawberries, washed and dried
- 1/4 cup dark chocolate, melted

Instructions:
1. Dip each strawberry into melted dark chocolate, covering half the strawberry.
2. Place on parchment paper and allow the chocolate to set.
3. Enjoy this sweet treat with the goodness of dark chocolate and strawberries.

Chapter 2: Lunchtime Delights

1. Salmon and Quinoa Salad

Ingredients:
- 1 cup cooked quinoa
- 4 ounces grilled salmon
- 1 cup mixed greens
- 1/2 cucumber, sliced
- Cherry tomatoes, halved
- 2 tablespoons olive oil
- 1 tablespoon balsamic vinegar
- Salt and pepper to taste

Instructions:
1. In a bowl, combine cooked quinoa, mixed greens, cucumber, and cherry tomatoes.
2. Top with grilled salmon.
3. Drizzle with olive oil and balsamic vinegar.
4. Season with salt and pepper. Toss gently and enjoy.

---

2. Vegetarian Chickpea and Spinach Stew

Ingredients:
- 1 can chickpeas, drained
- 2 cups fresh spinach
- 1 onion, diced
- 2 cloves garlic, minced

- 1 can diced tomatoes
- 1 teaspoon cumin
- 1 teaspoon paprika
- Salt and pepper to taste

Instructions:
1. In a pot, sauté onions and garlic until softened.
2. Add chickpeas, diced tomatoes, cumin, paprika, salt, and pepper.
3. Simmer for 15-20 minutes.
4. Stir in fresh spinach until wilted. Serve hot.

---

3. Grilled Chicken and Avocado Wrap

Ingredients:
- 4 ounces grilled chicken breast, sliced
- 1 whole-grain wrap
- 1/2 avocado, sliced
- 1/4 cup shredded lettuce
- 2 tablespoons Greek yogurt
- Salt and pepper to taste

Instructions:
1. Lay the wrap flat and layer with sliced grilled chicken.
2. Add sliced avocado, shredded lettuce, and a dollop of Greek yogurt.
3. Season with salt and pepper.
4. Roll up the wrap and enjoy this protein-packed lunch.

---

4. Mediterranean Quinoa Bowl

Ingredients:
- 1 cup cooked quinoa
- 1/2 cup cherry tomatoes, halved
- 1/4 cup Kalamata olives, sliced
- 1/4 cup feta cheese, crumbled
- 1/4 cup cucumber, diced
- 2 tablespoons olive oil
- Fresh lemon juice, to taste
- Fresh basil, chopped
- Salt and pepper to taste

Instructions:
1. In a bowl, combine cooked quinoa, cherry tomatoes, Kalamata olives, feta cheese, and cucumber.
2. Drizzle with olive oil and fresh lemon juice.
3. Add chopped fresh basil.
4. Season with salt and pepper. Toss gently and serve.

---

5. Tofu and Vegetable Stir-Fry

Ingredients:
- 1 cup firm tofu, cubed
- 1 cup broccoli florets
- 1/2 cup bell peppers, sliced
- 1/4 cup carrots, julienned

- 2 tablespoons soy sauce
- 1 tablespoon sesame oil
- 1 teaspoon ginger, minced
- 1 clove garlic, minced

Instructions:
1. In a wok or skillet, heat sesame oil over medium-high heat.
2. Add minced ginger and garlic, stir-fry for 30 seconds.
3. Add tofu cubes and cook until golden brown.
4. Add broccoli, bell peppers, and carrots. Stir-fry until vegetables are tender-crisp.
5. Pour in soy sauce and toss to combine.
6. Serve hot over brown rice or quinoa.

---

6. Sweet Potato and Black Bean Salad

Ingredients:
- 2 cups sweet potatoes, roasted and diced
- 1 can black beans, drained
- 1/4 cup red onion, finely chopped
- 1/4 cup cilantro, chopped
- 1 lime, juiced
- 2 tablespoons olive oil
- Salt and pepper to taste

Instructions:
1. In a bowl, combine roasted sweet potatoes, black beans, red onion, and cilantro.
2. Drizzle with lime juice and olive oil.

3. Season with salt and pepper. Toss gently and enjoy.

---

7. Eggplant and Tomato Caprese

Ingredients:
- 1 large eggplant, sliced
- 1 cup cherry tomatoes, halved
- 1/2 cup fresh mozzarella, sliced
- Fresh basil leaves
- 2 tablespoons balsamic glaze
- Olive oil for grilling
- Salt and pepper to taste

Instructions:
1. Brush eggplant slices with olive oil and grill until tender.
2. On a serving platter, layer grilled eggplant, cherry tomatoes, and fresh mozzarella.
3. Garnish with fresh basil leaves.
4. Drizzle with balsamic glaze.
5. Season with salt and pepper. Serve as a refreshing caprese salad.

---

8. Lentil and Vegetable Soup

Ingredients:
- 1 cup cooked lentils
- 1/2 cup carrots, diced

- 1/2 cup celery, diced
- 1/2 cup zucchini, diced
- 1 onion, diced
- 2 cloves garlic, minced
- 4 cups vegetable broth
- 1 teaspoon cumin
- 1 teaspoon thyme
- Salt and pepper to taste

Instructions:
1. In a pot, sauté onions and garlic until softened.
2. Add carrots, celery, zucchini, cooked lentils, vegetable broth, cumin, thyme, salt, and pepper.
3. Simmer for 20-25 minutes until vegetables are tender. Serve hot.

---

9. Quinoa and Chickpea Buddha Bowl

Ingredients:
- 1 cup cooked quinoa
- 1/2 cup chickpeas, cooked
- 1/2 cup cherry tomatoes, halved
- 1/4 cup cucumber, diced
- 1/4 cup hummus
- 2 tablespoons tahini dressing
- Fresh parsley, chopped
- Salt and pepper to taste

Instructions:

1. In a bowl, arrange cooked quinoa, chickpeas, cherry tomatoes, and diced cucumber.
2. Add dollops of hummus and drizzle with tahini dressing.
3. Garnish with fresh parsley.
4. Season with salt and pepper. Enjoy this nourishing Buddha bowl.

---

10. Chicken and

Vegetable Brown Rice Bowl

Ingredients:
- 4 ounces grilled chicken breast, sliced
- 1 cup cooked brown rice
- 1/2 cup broccoli florets
- 1/2 cup bell peppers, sliced
- 2 tablespoons soy sauce
- 1 tablespoon olive oil
- 1 teaspoon ginger, minced
- 1 clove garlic, minced

Instructions:
1. In a pan, heat olive oil over medium-high heat.
2. Add minced ginger and garlic, stir briefly.
3. Add sliced chicken, broccoli, and bell peppers. Cook until vegetables are tender.
4. Pour in soy sauce and toss to combine.
5. Serve over cooked brown rice.

---

11. Turkey and Cranberry Wrap

Ingredients:
- 4 ounces sliced turkey breast
- 1 whole-grain wrap
- 2 tablespoons cranberry sauce
- 1/4 cup baby spinach
- 1/4 cup shredded carrots
- Salt and pepper to taste

Instructions:
1. Lay the wrap flat and layer with sliced turkey.
2. Spread cranberry sauce over the turkey.
3. Add baby spinach and shredded carrots.
4. Season with salt and pepper.
5. Roll up the wrap and enjoy this festive and satisfying lunch.

---

12. Chickpea and Quinoa Stuffed Bell Peppers

Ingredients:
- 1 cup cooked quinoa
- 1 can chickpeas, drained
- 4 bell peppers, halved
- 1/2 cup cherry tomatoes, diced
- 1/4 cup red onion, finely chopped
- 2 tablespoons olive oil

- 1 teaspoon cumin
- 1 teaspoon smoked paprika
- Salt and pepper to taste

Instructions:
1. Preheat the oven to 375°F (190°C).
2. In a bowl, combine cooked quinoa, chickpeas, cherry tomatoes, red onion, olive oil, cumin, smoked paprika, salt, and pepper.
3. Stuff the bell peppers with the mixture.
4. Bake for 25-30 minutes or until the peppers are tender.

---

13. Miso-Glazed Salmon with Brown Rice

Ingredients:
- 4 ounces salmon fillet
- 1 cup cooked brown rice
- 2 tablespoons miso paste
- 1 tablespoon soy sauce
- 1 tablespoon honey
- 1 teaspoon ginger, minced
- 1 clove garlic, minced

Instructions:
1. Preheat the oven to 400°F (200°C).
2. In a small bowl, mix miso paste, soy sauce, honey, minced ginger, and minced garlic.
3. Brush the miso glaze over the salmon fillet.
4. Bake for 15-20 minutes or until the salmon is cooked through.
5. Serve over a bed of cooked brown rice.

---

14. Spinach and Feta Stuffed Chicken Breast

Ingredients:
- 2 boneless, skinless chicken breasts
- 1 cup fresh spinach, chopped
- 1/4 cup feta cheese, crumbled
- 1 tablespoon olive oil
- 1 teaspoon Italian seasoning
- Salt and pepper to taste

Instructions:
1. Preheat the oven to 375°F (190°C).
2. Butterfly the chicken breasts.
3. In a bowl, mix chopped spinach, feta cheese, olive oil, Italian seasoning, salt, and pepper.
4. Stuff each chicken breast with the spinach and feta mixture.
5. Bake for 25-30 minutes or until the chicken is cooked through.

---

15. Quinoa and Black Bean Salad Bowl

Ingredients:
- 1 cup cooked quinoa
- 1 can black beans, drained
- 1/2 cup corn kernels
- 1/4 cup red bell pepper, diced
- 2 tablespoons lime juice

- 1 tablespoon olive oil
- Fresh cilantro, chopped
- Salt and pepper to taste

Instructions:
1. In a bowl, combine cooked quinoa, black beans, corn, and diced red bell pepper.
2. Drizzle with lime juice and olive oil.
3. Add chopped fresh cilantro.
4. Season with salt and pepper. Toss gently and enjoy this flavorful salad bowl.

---

16. Tomato Basil and Mozzarella Caprese Wrap

Ingredients:
- 1 whole-grain wrap
- 1 large tomato, sliced
- Fresh mozzarella cheese, sliced
- Fresh basil leaves
- 1 tablespoon balsamic glaze
- Salt and pepper to taste

Instructions:
1. Lay the wrap flat and layer with sliced tomatoes, mozzarella, and fresh basil leaves.
2. Drizzle with balsamic glaze.
3. Season with salt and pepper.
4. Roll up the wrap and savor this classic Caprese combination.

---

17. Shrimp and Broccoli Stir-Fry

Ingredients:
- 1 cup shrimp, peeled and deveined
- 1 cup broccoli florets
- 1/2 cup snap peas
- 1/4 cup carrots, julienned
- 2 tablespoons soy sauce
- 1 tablespoon hoisin sauce
- 1 tablespoon sesame oil
- 1 teaspoon garlic, minced
- 1 teaspoon ginger, minced

Instructions:
1. In a wok or skillet, heat sesame oil over medium-high heat.
2. Add minced garlic and ginger, stir-fry for 30 seconds.
3. Add shrimp, broccoli, snap peas, and julienned carrots.
4. Pour in soy sauce and hoisin sauce. Toss to combine.
5. Cook until shrimp are pink and vegetables are crisp-tender.

---

18. Mushroom and Barley Soup

Ingredients:
- 1 cup cooked barley
- 1 cup mushrooms, sliced
- 1/2 cup celery, diced
- 1/2 cup carrots, diced

- 1 onion, diced
- 2 cloves garlic, minced
- 4 cups vegetable broth
- 1 teaspoon thyme
- Salt and pepper to taste

Instructions:
1. In a pot, sauté onions and garlic until softened.
2. Add mushrooms, celery, carrots, cooked barley, vegetable broth, thyme, salt, and pepper.
3. Simmer for 20-25 minutes until vegetables are tender. Serve hot.

---

19. Chickpea and Veggie Wrap

Ingredients:
- 1 whole-grain wrap
- 1 can chickpeas, mashed
- 1/4 cup cucumber, diced
- 1/4 cup red onion, finely chopped
- 2 tablespoons hummus
- Fresh parsley, chopped
- Salt and pepper to taste

Instructions:
1. Lay the wrap flat and spread mashed chickpeas over it.
2. Add diced cucumber, chopped red onion, and dollops of hummus.
3. Sprinkle with fresh parsley.

4. Season with salt and pepper.
5. Roll up the wrap and enjoy this plant-based delight.

---

20. Cauliflower and Chickpea Curry

Ingredients:
- 1 cup cauliflower florets
- 1 can chickpeas, drained
- 1/2 cup tomatoes, diced
- 1/4 cup coconut milk
- 1 tablespoon curry powder
- 1 teaspoon turmeric
- 1 teaspoon cumin
- Salt and pepper to taste

Instructions:
1. In a pan, combine cauliflower, chickpeas, diced tomatoes, coconut milk, curry powder, turmeric, cumin, salt, and pepper.
2. Simmer until cauliflower is tender and the curry is flavorful.
3. Serve over rice or quinoa.

---

21. Mediterranean Chickpea Salad

Ingredients:
- 1 can chickpeas, drained
- 1 cup cucumber, diced
- 1 cup cherry tomatoes, halved

- 1/4 cup red onion, finely chopped
- 1/4 cup feta cheese, crumbled
- 2 tablespoons olive oil
- 1 tablespoon lemon juice
- Fresh oregano, chopped
- Salt and pepper to taste

Instructions:
1. In a bowl, combine chickpeas, cucumber, cherry tomatoes, red onion, and feta cheese.
2. Drizzle with olive oil and lemon juice.
3. Add fresh oregano.
4. Season with salt and pepper. Toss gently and enjoy this refreshing Mediterranean salad.

---

22. Chicken Caesar Salad Wrap

Ingredients:
- 4 ounces grilled chicken breast, sliced
- 1 whole-grain wrap
- 1 cup romaine lettuce, chopped
- 2 tablespoons Caesar dressing
- 1/4 cup croutons
- Parmesan cheese, grated

Instructions:
1. Lay the wrap flat and layer with sliced grilled chicken.
2. Add chopped romaine lettuce.
3. Drizzle with Caesar dressing.

4. Sprinkle croutons and grated Parmesan cheese.
5. Roll up the wrap for a satisfying Caesar salad on the go.

---

23. Stuffed Bell Peppers with Turkey and Quinoa

Ingredients:
- 4 bell peppers, halved
- 1 cup cooked quinoa
- 1/2 pound ground turkey
- 1/2 cup black beans, drained
- 1/2 cup corn kernels
- 1/4 cup salsa
- 1 teaspoon cumin
- 1 teaspoon chili powder
- Salt and pepper to taste

Instructions:
1. Preheat the oven to 375°F (190°C).
2. In a pan, cook ground turkey until browned.
3. In a bowl, mix cooked quinoa, browned turkey, black beans, corn, salsa, cumin, chili powder, salt, and pepper.
4. Stuff bell peppers with the mixture.
5. Bake for 25-30 minutes or until peppers are tender.

—

24. Spaghetti Squash Primavera

Ingredients:
- 1 spaghetti squash, cooked and shredded
- 1 cup cherry tomatoes, halved
- 1/2 cup broccoli florets
- 1/4 cup black olives, sliced
- 1/4 cup Parmesan cheese, grated
- 2 tablespoons olive oil
- 1 teaspoon Italian seasoning
- Salt and pepper to taste

Instructions:
1. In a pan, sauté cherry tomatoes, broccoli, and black olives in olive oil.
2. Add shredded spaghetti squash and toss until heated through.
3. Sprinkle with Parmesan cheese and Italian seasoning.
4. Season with salt and pepper. Serve warm.

---

25. Quinoa and Lentil Patties

Ingredients:
- 1 cup cooked quinoa
- 1 cup cooked lentils
- 1/2 cup breadcrumbs
- 1/4 cup onion, finely chopped
- 1 egg
- 1 teaspoon cumin
- 1 teaspoon coriander

- Salt and pepper to taste
- Olive oil for cooking

Instructions:
1. In a bowl, combine cooked quinoa, cooked lentils, breadcrumbs, chopped onion, egg, cumin, coriander, salt, and pepper.
2. Form into patties.
3. Heat olive oil in a skillet and cook patties until golden brown on each side.
4. Serve with a side salad for a wholesome lunch.

---

26. Asian-Inspired Tofu and Vegetable Stir-Fry

Ingredients:
- 1 cup tofu, cubed
- 1 cup broccoli florets
- 1/2 cup snap peas
- 1/4 cup carrots, julienned
- 2 tablespoons soy sauce
- 1 tablespoon hoisin sauce
- 1 tablespoon sesame oil
- 1 teaspoon ginger, minced
- 1 teaspoon garlic, minced

Instructions:
1. In a wok or skillet, heat sesame oil over medium-high heat.
2. Add minced ginger and garlic, stir-fry for 30 seconds.
3. Add tofu cubes, broccoli, snap peas, and julienned carrots.
4. Pour in soy sauce and hoisin sauce. Toss to combine.

5. Cook until tofu is golden and vegetables are crisp-tender.

---

27. Broccoli and Cheddar Stuffed Baked Potatoes

Ingredients:
- 4 medium-sized baked potatoes
- 1 cup broccoli, steamed and chopped
- 1/2 cup cheddar cheese, shredded
- 1/4 cup Greek yogurt
- 2 tablespoons chives, chopped
- Salt and pepper to taste

Instructions:
1. Cut a slit in each baked potato and fluff the insides with a fork.
2. In a bowl, mix steamed broccoli, cheddar cheese, Greek yogurt, chives, salt, and pepper.
3. Stuff each baked potato with the broccoli and cheddar mixture.
4. Bake for an additional 10 minutes or until cheese is melted.

---

28. Egg Drop Soup with Spinach and Mushrooms

Ingredients:
- 4 cups chicken or vegetable broth
- 2 eggs, beaten
- 1 cup spinach leaves
- 1 cup mushrooms, sliced
- 1 tablespoon soy sauce

- 1 teaspoon sesame oil
- Green onions, chopped

Instructions:
1. In a pot, bring chicken or vegetable broth to a simmer.
2. Add mushrooms and spinach, cook until tender.
3. Slowly pour beaten eggs into the simmering broth, stirring gently.
4. Add soy sauce and sesame oil.
5. Garnish with chopped green onions. Serve hot.

---

29. Cajun Shrimp and Quinoa Skillet

Ingredients:
- 1 cup cooked quinoa
- 1/2 pound shrimp, peeled and deveined
- 1 cup bell peppers, sliced
- 1/2 cup red onion, sliced
- 2 tablespoons Cajun seasoning
- 1 tablespoon olive oil
- Fresh parsley, chopped
- Lemon wedges for serving

Instructions:
1. In a skillet, heat olive oil over medium-high heat.
2. Add shrimp, bell peppers, and red onion.
3. Sprinkle with Cajun seasoning and cook until shrimp are pink and vegetables are tender.
4. Stir in cooked quinoa.

5. Garnish with fresh parsley and serve with lemon wedges.

---

30. Caprese Quinoa Bowl

Ingredients:
- 1 cup cooked quinoa
- 1 cup cherry tomatoes, halved
- Fresh mozzarella balls
- Fresh basil leaves
- 2 tablespoons balsamic glaze
- Olive oil
- Salt and pepper to taste

Instructions:
1. In a bowl, combine cooked quinoa, cherry tomatoes, fresh mozzarella balls, and fresh basil leaves.
2. Drizzle with balsamic glaze and olive oil.
3. Season with salt and pepper. Toss gently and savor this Caprese-inspired quinoa bowl.

Chapter 3: Dinner for Bone Health

1. Grilled Salmon with Lemon-Dill Sauce

Ingredients:
- 4 salmon fillets
- 1 lemon, juiced
- 2 tablespoons fresh dill, chopped
- 2 cloves garlic, minced
- 1 tablespoon olive oil
- Salt and pepper to taste

Instructions:
1. Preheat the grill.
2. In a bowl, mix lemon juice, chopped dill, minced garlic, olive oil, salt, and pepper.
3. Brush the mixture over salmon fillets.
4. Grill for 5-7 minutes per side or until cooked through. Serve with your favorite roasted vegetables.

---

2. Quinoa-Stuffed Bell Peppers

Ingredients:
- 4 bell peppers, halved
- 1 cup cooked quinoa
- 1 can black beans, drained
- 1 cup corn kernels
- 1/2 cup diced tomatoes

- 1 teaspoon cumin
- 1 teaspoon chili powder
- Salt and pepper to taste
- Shredded cheese for topping (optional)

Instructions:
1. Preheat the oven to 375°F (190°C).
2. In a bowl, mix cooked quinoa, black beans, corn, diced tomatoes, cumin, chili powder, salt, and pepper.
3. Stuff bell pepper halves with the quinoa mixture.
4. Bake for 25-30 minutes or until peppers are tender.
5. If desired, sprinkle with shredded cheese before serving.

---

3. Baked Chicken Thighs with Rosemary and Garlic

Ingredients:
- 4 chicken thighs, bone-in, skin-on
- 2 tablespoons olive oil
- 2 tablespoons fresh rosemary, chopped
- 4 cloves garlic, minced
- Salt and pepper to taste

Instructions:
1. Preheat the oven to 400°F (200°C).
2. In a bowl, mix olive oil, chopped rosemary, minced garlic, salt, and pepper.
3. Rub the mixture over chicken thighs.
4. Bake for 30-35 minutes or until the chicken reaches an internal temperature of 165°F (74°C).

5. Serve with roasted sweet potatoes or steamed broccoli.

---

4. Vegetarian Lentil and Vegetable Stir-Fry

Ingredients:
- 1 cup cooked lentils
- 1 cup broccoli florets
- 1/2 cup bell peppers, sliced
- 1/4 cup carrots, julienned
- 2 tablespoons soy sauce
- 1 tablespoon hoisin sauce
- 1 tablespoon sesame oil
- 1 teaspoon ginger, minced
- 1 teaspoon garlic, minced

Instructions:
1. In a wok or skillet, heat sesame oil over medium-high heat.
2. Add minced ginger and garlic, stir-fry for 30 seconds.
3. Add cooked lentils, broccoli, bell peppers, and julienned carrots.
4. Pour in soy sauce and hoisin sauce. Toss to combine.
5. Cook until vegetables are crisp-tender. Serve over brown rice.

---

5. Sweet Potato and Chickpea Curry

Ingredients:
- 2 sweet potatoes, peeled and diced

- 1 can chickpeas, drained
- 1 cup coconut milk
- 1 onion, diced
- 2 cloves garlic, minced
- 1 tablespoon curry powder
- 1 teaspoon turmeric
- 1 teaspoon cumin
- Salt and pepper to taste
- Fresh cilantro for garnish

Instructions:
1. In a pot, sauté onions and garlic until softened.
2. Add diced sweet potatoes, chickpeas, coconut milk, curry powder, turmeric, cumin, salt, and pepper.
3. Simmer for 20-25 minutes or until sweet potatoes are tender.
4. Garnish with fresh cilantro before serving. Serve over basmati rice.

---

6. Mushroom and Spinach Stuffed Chicken Breast

Ingredients:
- 4 boneless, skinless chicken breasts
- 1 cup mushrooms, finely chopped
- 1 cup fresh spinach, chopped
- 1/2 cup feta cheese, crumbled
- 2 tablespoons olive oil
- 1 teaspoon Italian seasoning
- Salt and pepper to taste

Instructions:
1. Preheat the oven to 375°F (190°C).
2. In a pan, sauté mushrooms and spinach in olive oil until wilted.
3. Stir in crumbled feta cheese, Italian seasoning, salt, and pepper.
4. Cut a pocket into each chicken breast and stuff with the mushroom and spinach mixture.
5. Bake for 25-30 minutes or until the chicken is cooked through.

---

7. Baked Cod with Mediterranean Salsa

Ingredients:
- 4 cod fillets
- 1 cup cherry tomatoes, halved
- 1/2 cup Kalamata olives, sliced
- 1/4 cup red onion, finely chopped
- 2 tablespoons fresh parsley, chopped
- 1 tablespoon olive oil
- 1 lemon, juiced
- Salt and pepper to taste

Instructions:
1. Preheat the oven to 400°F (200°C).
2. Place cod fillets on a baking sheet.
3. In a bowl, mix cherry tomatoes, Kalamata olives, red onion, fresh parsley, olive oil, lemon juice, salt, and pepper.
4. Spoon the Mediterranean salsa over the cod fillets.
5. Bake for 15-20 minutes or until the fish flakes easily with a fork.

---

8. Chickpea and Vegetable Curry

Ingredients:
- 1 can chickpeas, drained
- 1 cup cauliflower florets
- 1/2 cup peas
- 1/2 cup carrots, diced
- 1 onion, diced
- 2 cloves garlic, minced
- 1 can diced tomatoes
- 1 cup vegetable broth
- 1 tablespoon curry powder
- 1 teaspoon turmeric
- Salt and pepper to taste

Instructions:
1. In a pot, sauté onions and garlic until softened.
2. Add chickpeas, cauliflower, peas, carrots, diced tomatoes, vegetable broth, curry powder, turmeric, salt, and pepper.
3. Simmer for 20-25 minutes until vegetables are tender. Serve over basmati rice.

---

9. Shrimp and Broccoli Quinoa Bowl

Ingredients:
- 1 cup cooked quinoa
- 1 cup shrimp, peeled and deveined
- 1 cup broccoli florets

- 1/2 cup bell peppers, sliced
- 2 tablespoons soy sauce
- 1 tablespoon hoisin sauce
- 1 tablespoon sesame oil
- 1 teaspoon ginger, minced
- 1 teaspoon garlic, minced

Instructions:
1. In a wok or skillet, heat sesame oil over medium-high heat.
2. Add minced ginger and garlic, stir-fry for 30 seconds.
3. Add shrimp, broccoli, bell peppers, and cooked quinoa.
4. Pour in soy sauce and hoisin sauce. Toss to combine.
5. Cook until shrimp are pink and vegetables are crisp-tender.

---

10. Eggplant Parmesan with Whole-Grain Pasta

Ingredients:
- 1 large eggplant, sliced
- 2 cups whole-grain pasta, cooked
- 2 cups marinara sauce
- 1 cup mozzarella cheese, shredded
- 1/4 cup Parmesan cheese, grated
- Fresh basil leaves for garnish
- Olive oil for baking

Instructions:
1. Preheat the oven to 375°F (190°C).
2. Brush eggplant slices with olive oil and bake until tender.

3. In a baking dish, layer cooked whole-grain pasta, marinara sauce, baked eggplant slices, and cheeses.
4. Repeat the layers and finish with a layer of cheese on top.
5. Bake for 25-30 minutes or until the cheese is melted and bubbly.
6. Garnish with fresh basil leaves before serving.

---

11. Lemon Garlic Herb Grilled Chicken

Ingredients:
- 4 boneless, skinless chicken breasts
- Zest and juice of 2 lemons
- 3 cloves garlic, minced
- 2 tablespoons fresh herbs (rosemary, thyme, or oregano), chopped
- 2 tablespoons olive oil
- Salt and pepper to taste

Instructions:
1. In a bowl, mix lemon zest, lemon juice, minced garlic, chopped herbs, olive oil, salt, and pepper.
2. Marinate chicken breasts in the mixture for at least 30 minutes.
3. Grill until cooked through, about 6-8 minutes per side. Serve with steamed vegetables.

—

12. Turkey and Vegetable Quinoa Bowl

Ingredients:
- 1 cup cooked quinoa
- 1/2 pound ground turkey
- 1 cup mixed vegetables (carrots, peas, corn)
- 1/4 cup soy sauce
- 2 tablespoons sesame oil
- 1 teaspoon ginger, minced
- 1 teaspoon garlic, minced
- Green onions for garnish

Instructions:
1. In a skillet, cook ground turkey until browned.
2. Add mixed vegetables, soy sauce, sesame oil, minced ginger, and minced garlic.
3. Stir-fry until vegetables are tender. Serve over cooked quinoa.
4. Garnish with chopped green onions.

---

13. Roasted Vegetable and Chickpea Salad

Ingredients:
- 1 can chickpeas, drained
- 2 cups mixed vegetables (zucchini, bell peppers, cherry tomatoes)
- 2 tablespoons olive oil
- 1 teaspoon cumin
- 1 teaspoon smoked paprika
- Salt and pepper to taste

- Fresh parsley for garnish

Instructions:
1. Preheat the oven to 400°F (200°C).
2. Toss chickpeas and mixed vegetables with olive oil, cumin, smoked paprika, salt, and pepper.
3. Roast for 25-30 minutes or until vegetables are caramelized.
4. Garnish with fresh parsley before serving.

---

14. Salmon and Asparagus Foil Packets

Ingredients:
- 4 salmon fillets
- 1 bunch asparagus, trimmed
- 2 tablespoons lemon juice
- 2 tablespoons Dijon mustard
- 2 cloves garlic, minced
- 2 tablespoons fresh dill, chopped
- Salt and pepper to taste

Instructions:
1. Preheat the oven to 400°F (200°C).
2. In a bowl, mix lemon juice, Dijon mustard, minced garlic, chopped dill, salt, and pepper.
3. Place each salmon fillet on a piece of foil, surround with asparagus, and spoon the sauce over.
4. Seal the foil packets and bake for 15-20 minutes. Serve over brown rice.

---

15. Chickpea and Spinach Coconut Curry

Ingredients:
- 1 can chickpeas, drained
- 2 cups fresh spinach
- 1 onion, diced
- 2 cloves garlic, minced
- 1 can coconut milk
- 1 tablespoon curry powder
- 1 teaspoon turmeric
- 1 teaspoon cumin
- Salt and pepper to taste

Instructions:
1. In a pot, sauté onions and garlic until softened.
2. Add chickpeas, fresh spinach, coconut milk, curry powder, turmeric, cumin, salt, and pepper.
3. Simmer for 15-20 minutes until flavors meld. Serve over basmati rice.

---

16. Stuffed Portobello Mushrooms with Quinoa and Kale

Ingredients:
- 4 large portobello mushrooms
- 1 cup cooked quinoa
- 1 cup kale, chopped
- 1/4 cup sun-dried tomatoes, chopped

- 1/4 cup feta cheese, crumbled
- 2 tablespoons balsamic glaze
- 2 tablespoons olive oil
- Salt and pepper to taste

Instructions:
1. Preheat the oven to 375°F (190°C).
2. Remove the stems from portobello mushrooms and brush with olive oil.
3. In a bowl, mix cooked quinoa, chopped kale, sun-dried tomatoes, crumbled feta, salt, and pepper.
4. Stuff each mushroom cap with the quinoa mixture.
5. Bake for 20-25 minutes. Drizzle with balsamic glaze before serving.

---

17. Sesame Ginger Tofu Stir-Fry

Ingredients:
- 1 cup tofu, cubed
- 1 cup broccoli florets
- 1/2 cup snap peas
- 1/4 cup carrots, julienned
- 2 tablespoons soy sauce
- 1 tablespoon hoisin sauce
- 1 tablespoon sesame oil
- 1 teaspoon ginger, minced
- 1 teaspoon garlic, minced

Instructions:

1. In a wok or skillet, heat sesame oil over medium-high heat.
2.

 Add minced ginger and garlic, stir-fry for 30 seconds.
3. Add tofu cubes, broccoli, snap peas, and julienned carrots.
4. Pour in soy sauce and hoisin sauce. Toss to combine.
5. Cook until tofu is golden and vegetables are crisp-tender. Serve over brown rice.

---

18. Miso-Glazed Eggplant with Brown Rice

Ingredients:
- 2 eggplants, sliced
- 1 cup cooked brown rice
- 2 tablespoons miso paste
- 1 tablespoon soy sauce
- 1 tablespoon honey
- 1 teaspoon sesame oil
- 1 teaspoon ginger, minced

Instructions:
1. Preheat the oven to 400°F (200°C).
2. In a bowl, mix miso paste, soy sauce, honey, sesame oil, and minced ginger.
3. Brush the miso glaze over eggplant slices.
4. Roast for 20-25 minutes or until eggplant is tender. Serve over brown rice.

---

19. Cauliflower and Chickpea Masala

Ingredients:
- 1 cup cauliflower florets
- 1 can chickpeas, drained
- 1 cup tomatoes, diced
- 1/2 cup onion, diced
- 2 cloves garlic, minced
- 1/4 cup coconut milk
- 1 tablespoon curry powder
- 1 teaspoon turmeric
- 1 teaspoon cumin
- Salt and pepper to taste

Instructions:
1. In a pan, sauté onions and garlic until softened.
2. Add cauliflower, chickpeas, diced tomatoes, coconut milk, curry powder, turmeric, cumin, salt, and pepper.
3. Simmer for 15-20 minutes until cauliflower is tender. Serve with quinoa.

---

20. Lemon Herb Baked Cod

Ingredients:
- 4 cod fillets
- 1 lemon, juiced
- 2 tablespoons fresh parsley, chopped
- 2 tablespoons olive oil

- 2 cloves garlic, minced
- Salt and pepper to taste

Instructions:
1. Preheat the oven to 375°F (190°C).
2. Place cod fillets in a baking dish.
3. In a bowl, mix lemon juice, chopped parsley, olive oil, minced garlic, salt, and pepper.
4. Pour the mixture over the cod fillets.
5. Bake for 15-20 minutes or until the fish flakes easily with a fork.

---

21. Garlic Rosemary Roasted Pork Tenderloin

Ingredients:
- 2 pork tenderloins
- 3 cloves garlic, minced
- 2 tablespoons fresh rosemary, chopped
- 2 tablespoons olive oil
- Salt and pepper to taste

Instructions:
1. Preheat the oven to 400°F (200°C).
2. In a bowl, mix minced garlic, chopped rosemary, olive oil, salt, and pepper.
3. Rub the mixture over the pork tenderloins.
4. Roast for 25-30 minutes or until the internal temperature reaches 145°F (63°C).
5. Let it rest for 5 minutes before slicing.

---

22. Vegetarian Lentil Shepherd's Pie

Ingredients:
- 2 cups cooked lentils
- 1 cup mixed vegetables (peas, carrots, corn)
- 1 onion, diced
- 2 cloves garlic, minced
- 1 cup vegetable broth
- 2 tablespoons tomato paste
- 2 tablespoons Worcestershire sauce
- Mashed sweet potatoes for topping

Instructions:
1. In a pan, sauté onions and garlic until softened.
2. Add cooked lentils, mixed vegetables, vegetable broth, tomato paste, and Worcestershire sauce.
3. Simmer until the mixture thickens.
4. Spoon the lentil mixture into a baking dish and top with mashed sweet potatoes.
5. Bake for 20-25 minutes or until the top is golden brown.

---

23. Teriyaki Glazed Salmon with Broccoli

Ingredients:
- 4 salmon fillets
- 1 cup broccoli florets
- 1/4 cup low-sodium teriyaki sauce

- 2 tablespoons honey
- 1 tablespoon sesame oil
- 1 teaspoon ginger, minced
- 1 teaspoon garlic, minced

Instructions:
1. Preheat the oven to 400°F (200°C).
2. In a bowl, mix teriyaki sauce, honey, sesame oil, minced ginger, and minced garlic.
3. Place salmon fillets and broccoli on a baking sheet.
4. Brush the teriyaki mixture over salmon and broccoli.
5. Bake for 15-20 minutes or until the salmon is cooked through.

---

24. Mushroom and Spinach Quiche with Whole-Grain Crust

Ingredients:
- 1 whole-grain pie crust
- 1 cup mushrooms, sliced
- 2 cups fresh spinach
- 1/2 cup feta cheese, crumbled
- 4 eggs
- 1 cup milk
- Salt and pepper to taste

Instructions:
1. Preheat the oven to 375°F (190°C).
2. In a pan, sauté mushrooms until browned.
3. Add fresh spinach and sauté until wilted.

4. Line a pie crust with the mushroom and spinach mixture. Sprinkle feta cheese on top.
5. In a bowl, whisk together eggs, milk, salt, and pepper. Pour over the vegetables and cheese.
6. Bake for 30-35 minutes or until the quiche is set.

---

25. Honey Mustard Glazed Chicken with Roasted Vegetables

Ingredients:
- 4 chicken thighs, bone-in, skin-on
- 1 cup baby potatoes, halved
- 1 cup baby carrots
- 2 tablespoons Dijon mustard
- 2 tablespoons honey
- 1 tablespoon olive oil
- 1 teaspoon dried thyme
- Salt and pepper to taste

Instructions:
1. Preheat the oven to 400°F (200°C).
2. In a bowl, mix Dijon mustard, honey, olive oil, dried thyme, salt, and pepper.
3. Place chicken thighs, potatoes, and carrots on a baking sheet.
4. Brush the honey mustard mixture over the chicken and vegetables.
5. Roast for 35-40 minutes or until the chicken is cooked through.

---

26. Quinoa and Black Bean Stuffed Peppers

Ingredients:
- 4 bell peppers, halved
- 1 cup cooked quinoa
- 1 can black beans, drained
- 1 cup corn kernels
- 1 cup diced tomatoes
- 1 teaspoon cumin
- 1 teaspoon chili powder
- Salt and pepper to taste
- Shredded cheddar cheese for topping

Instructions:
1. Preheat the oven to 375°F (190°C).
2. In a bowl, mix cooked quinoa, black beans, corn, diced tomatoes, cumin, chili powder, salt, and pepper.
3. Stuff bell pepper halves with the quinoa mixture.
4. Top with shredded cheddar cheese.
5. Bake for 25-30 minutes or until peppers are tender.

---

27. Spicy Thai Basil Tofu Stir-Fry

Ingredients:
- 1 cup tofu, cubed
- 1 cup broccoli florets
- 1/2 cup bell peppers, sliced
- 1/4 cup snap peas
- 2 tablespoons soy sauce

- 1 tablespoon oyster sauce
- 1 tablespoon chili garlic sauce
- 1 teaspoon sesame oil
- 1 teaspoon ginger, minced
- 1 teaspoon garlic, minced

Instructions:
1. In a wok or skillet, heat sesame oil over medium-high heat.
2. Add minced ginger and garlic, stir-fry for 30 seconds.
3. Add tofu cubes, broccoli, bell peppers, and snap peas.
4. Pour in soy sauce, oyster sauce, and chili garlic sauce. Toss to combine.
5. Cook until tofu is golden and vegetables are crisp-tender.

---

28. Caprese Stuffed Chicken Breast

Ingredients:
- 4 chicken breasts, boneless, skinless
- 1 cup cherry tomatoes, halved
- Fresh mozzarella balls
- Fresh basil leaves
- Balsamic glaze
- Olive oil
- Salt and pepper to taste

Instructions:
1. Preheat the oven to 375°F (190°C).
2. Cut a pocket into each chicken breast.

3. Stuff with cherry tomatoes, mozzarella balls, and fresh basil leaves.
4. Drizzle with balsamic glaze and olive oil.
5. Season with salt and pepper. Bake for 25-30 minutes or until chicken is cooked through.

---

29. Mediterranean Chickpea Bowl

Ingredients:
- 1 cup cooked quinoa
- 1 can chickpeas, drained
- 1 cup cucumber, diced
- 1 cup cherry tomatoes, halved
- 1/4 cup red onion, finely chopped
- 1/4 cup feta cheese, crumbled
- Kalamata olives
- Olive oil
- Lemon juice
- Fresh oregano, chopped
- Salt and pepper to taste

Instructions:
1. In a bowl, combine cooked quinoa, chickpeas, cucumber, cherry tomatoes, red onion, feta cheese, and Kalamata olives.
2. Drizzle with olive oil and lemon juice.
3. Sprinkle with fresh oregano, salt, and pepper. Toss gently and enjoy!

---

30. Stuffed Acorn Squash with Wild Rice and Cranberries

Ingredients:
- 2 acorn squash, halved and seeds removed
- 1 cup wild rice, cooked
- 1/2 cup dried cranberries
- 1/4 cup pecans, chopped
- 2 tablespoons maple syrup
- 1 tablespoon olive oil
- Fresh thyme for garnish
- Salt and pepper to taste

Instructions:
1. Preheat the oven to 400°F (200°C).
2. Place acorn squash halves on a baking sheet.
3. In a bowl, mix cooked wild rice, dried cranberries, chopped pecans, maple syrup, olive oil, salt, and pepper.
4. Stuff each acorn squash half with the rice mixture.
5. Bake for 30-35 minutes or until squash is tender. Garnish with fresh thyme before serving.

Chapter 4: Snack Smart

1. Greek Yogurt Parfait

Ingredients:
- 1 cup Greek yogurt
- 1/2 cup granola
- 1/2 cup mixed berries
- Honey for drizzling

Instructions:
1. In a glass or bowl, layer Greek yogurt at the bottom.
2. Add a generous sprinkle of granola on top of the yogurt layer.
3. Top the granola with a mix of fresh berries, such as strawberries, blueberries, and raspberries.
4. Drizzle honey over the berries for added sweetness.
5. Repeat the layers as desired. Enjoy this calcium-rich Greek Yogurt Parfait!

---

2. Almond Butter and Banana Slices

Ingredients:
- Whole-grain crackers
- Almond butter
- Banana, sliced

Instructions:
1. Spread almond butter evenly on whole-grain crackers.

2. Place banana slices on top of the almond butter.
3. Serve and enjoy this magnesium-rich snack that combines the crunch of the crackers with the creaminess of almond butter and the sweetness of bananas.

---

3. Cheese and Whole Grain Crackers

Ingredients:
- Assorted cheese cubes (cheddar, mozzarella, etc.)
- Whole grain crackers

Instructions:
1. Arrange an assortment of cheese cubes on a plate.
2. Place a variety of whole-grain crackers next to the cheese.
3. Pair different cheeses with crackers for a delightful mix of flavors and textures.
4. Enjoy this calcium-rich cheese and cracker platter!

---

4. Dark Chocolate-Dipped Strawberries

Ingredients:
- Dark chocolate, melted
- Fresh strawberries

Instructions:
1. Melt dark chocolate in a heatproof bowl.

2. Dip fresh strawberries into the melted dark chocolate, coating them partially.
3. Place the dipped strawberries on a parchment paper-lined tray.
4. Allow the chocolate to set. Enjoy these magnesium-rich dark chocolate-dipped strawberries as a sweet treat.

---

5. Trail Mix with Nuts and Seeds

Ingredients:
- Almonds
- Walnuts
- Pumpkin seeds
- Dried apricots
- Dark chocolate chips

Instructions:
1. In a bowl, combine almonds, walnuts, pumpkin seeds, dried apricots (cut into bite-sized pieces), and dark chocolate chips.
2. Mix well to ensure an even distribution of ingredients.
3. Portion into snack-sized containers for a nutrient-packed trail mix.

---

6. Hummus and Veggie Sticks

Ingredients:
- Hummus (store-bought or homemade)
- Carrot sticks

- Cucumber slices
- Bell pepper strips

Instructions:
1. If using store-bought hummus, scoop it into a serving bowl. If making homemade hummus, follow your preferred recipe.
2. Wash and cut carrot sticks, cucumber slices, and bell pepper strips for dipping.
3. Arrange the veggie sticks around the hummus bowl.
4. Dip the veggies into the hummus and enjoy this calcium-rich and protein-packed snack.

---

7. Cottage Cheese with Pineapple Chunks

Ingredients:
- Cottage cheese
- Fresh pineapple chunks

Instructions:
1. Spoon cottage cheese into a bowl.
2. Add fresh pineapple chunks on top.
3. Mix gently or enjoy as a layered snack. Cottage cheese provides calcium, while pineapple adds a sweet and tangy flavor.

---

8. Kale Chips

Ingredients:

- Fresh kale leaves
- Olive oil
- Sea salt

Instructions:
1. Preheat the oven to 350°F (175°C).
2. Wash and thoroughly dry kale leaves. Remove stems and tear leaves into bite-sized pieces.
3. Toss kale pieces with a small amount of olive oil, ensuring each piece is lightly coated.
4. Spread kale on a baking sheet, ensuring they are in a single layer.
5. Sprinkle with sea salt.
6. Bake for 10-15 minutes or until crispy. Enjoy these calcium-rich kale chips!

---

9. Chia Seed Pudding

Ingredients:
- Chia seeds
- Almond milk
- Vanilla extract
- Mixed berries

Instructions:
1. In a bowl, mix chia seeds, almond milk, and a few drops of vanilla extract.
2. Stir well and refrigerate for at least two hours or overnight until it thickens.

3. Spoon the chia pudding into a glass or bowl.
4. Top with a variety of mixed berries for added flavor and antioxidants.

---

10. Apple Slices with Nut Butter

Ingredients:
- Apple slices
- Almond or peanut butter

Instructions:
1. Slice apples into thin wedges.
2. Spread almond or peanut butter on one side of each apple slice.
3. If desired, sprinkle with a touch of cinnamon for extra flavor.
4. Arrange the apple slices on a plate and enjoy this wholesome and satisfying snack.

These detailed instructions ensure that seniors over 60 can easily recreate these smart and bone-healthy snacks. Enjoy these flavorful and nutrient-packed options as part of your Bone-Healthy Cooking journey!Certainly! Here are the final 10 smart and bone-healthy snack ideas for your cookbook:

---

11. Avocado Toast with Tomato Slices

Ingredients:
- Whole-grain bread slices
- Ripe avocado
- Tomato, sliced
- Salt and pepper to taste

Instructions:
1. Toast whole-grain bread slices to your preference.
2. Mash ripe avocado and spread it over the toasted bread.
3. Top with fresh tomato slices.
4. Sprinkle with a pinch of salt and pepper.
5. Enjoy this snack rich in healthy fats, vitamins, and minerals.

---

12. Cucumber and Cream Cheese Roll-Ups

Ingredients:
- Cucumber, thinly sliced
- Cream cheese
- Smoked salmon (optional)
- Fresh dill for garnish

Instructions:
1. Lay cucumber slices flat.
2. Spread a thin layer of cream cheese on each slice.
3. Add a small piece of smoked salmon if desired.
4. Roll up the cucumber slices and secure with toothpicks.
5. Garnish with fresh dill before serving.

---

13. Mango Salsa with Whole-Grain Tortilla Chips

Ingredients:
- Ripe mango, diced
- Red onion, finely chopped
- Fresh cilantro, chopped
- Lime juice
- Whole-grain tortilla chips

Instructions:
1. In a bowl, combine diced mango, chopped red onion, and fresh cilantro.
2. Squeeze lime juice over the mixture and toss gently.
3. Serve with whole-grain tortilla chips for a tasty and vitamin C-rich snack.

---

14. Edamame with Sea Salt

Ingredients:
- Edamame (fresh or frozen)
- Sea salt

Instructions:
1. If using frozen edamame, steam or boil according to package instructions.
2. Sprinkle with sea salt before serving.
3. Enjoy these protein-packed edamame beans as a satisfying and calcium-rich snack.

---

15. Whole-Grain Crackers with Tuna Salad

Ingredients:
- Whole-grain crackers
- Canned tuna, drained
- Greek yogurt
- Celery, finely chopped
- Dill, chopped
- Salt and pepper to taste

Instructions:
1. In a bowl, mix drained tuna, Greek yogurt, chopped celery, and dill.
2. Season with salt and pepper to taste.
3. Spoon the tuna salad onto whole-grain crackers for a protein and calcium-rich snack.

---

16. Pumpkin Seeds and Dried Cranberries Mix

Ingredients:
- Pumpkin seeds (pepitas)
- Dried cranberries
- Dark chocolate chips

Instructions:

1. Combine pumpkin seeds, dried cranberries, and dark chocolate chips in a bowl.
2. Mix well to create a sweet and crunchy snack rich in magnesium and antioxidants.

---

17. Quinoa and Black Bean Stuffed Mini Peppers

Ingredients:
- Mini bell peppers, halved
- Cooked quinoa
- Black beans, canned and drained
- Cherry tomatoes, diced
- Feta cheese, crumbled

Instructions:
1. Fill mini bell pepper halves with cooked quinoa.
2. Top with black beans, diced cherry tomatoes, and crumbled feta.
3. Bake until peppers are tender for a delicious and nutrient-packed snack.

---

18. Cherry Tomatoes with Mozzarella Balls

Ingredients:
- Cherry tomatoes
- Fresh mozzarella balls
- Basil leaves

- Balsamic glaze

Instructions:
1. Thread cherry tomatoes, fresh mozzarella balls, and basil leaves onto toothpicks.
2. Arrange on a plate and drizzle with balsamic glaze.
3. Enjoy this refreshing and calcium-rich Caprese-inspired snack.

---

19. Sweet Potato Fries with Greek Yogurt Dip

Ingredients:
- Sweet potatoes, cut into fries
- Olive oil
- Paprika
- Greek yogurt
- Dijon mustard
- Garlic powder

Instructions:
1. Toss sweet potato fries with olive oil and a sprinkle of paprika.
2. Bake until crispy.
3. Mix Greek yogurt with Dijon mustard and garlic powder for a tasty dip.
4. Enjoy these vitamin A-rich sweet potato fries with a protein-packed dip.

---

20. Spinach and Feta Stuffed Mushrooms

Ingredients:
- Large mushrooms, cleaned and stems removed
- Fresh spinach, chopped
- Feta cheese, crumbled
- Garlic, minced
- Olive oil

Instructions:
1. Preheat the oven to 375°F (190°C).
2. In a pan, sauté chopped spinach and minced garlic in olive oil until wilted.
3. Fill mushroom caps with the spinach mixture and top with crumbled feta.
4. Bake until mushrooms are tender.
5. Enjoy these flavorful and calcium-rich stuffed mushrooms.

These detailed snack ideas offer a range of flavors and nutrients for bone health. Enjoy these smart snacks as part of your Bone-Healthy Cooking journey!Certainly! Here are the next 10 smart and bone-healthy snack ideas for your cookbook:

---

21. Blueberry and Almond Smoothie

Ingredients:
- 1 cup blueberries (fresh or frozen)
- 1 banana

- Almond milk
- Greek yogurt
- Almond butter

Instructions:
1. Blend blueberries, banana, a splash of almond milk, a spoonful of Greek yogurt, and a tablespoon of almond butter until smooth.
2. Pour into a glass and enjoy this antioxidant-rich smoothie for a nutrient-packed snack.

---

22. Whole-Grain Pita with Hummus and Cherry Tomatoes

Ingredients:
- Whole-grain pita bread
- Hummus
- Cherry tomatoes, halved
- Fresh parsley, chopped

Instructions:
1. Toast whole-grain pita bread.
2. Spread a layer of hummus on the pita.
3. Top with halved cherry tomatoes and sprinkle with fresh chopped parsley.
4. Slice and enjoy this fiber-rich and calcium-packed snack.

---

23. Apricot and Walnut Energy Bites

Ingredients:
- Dried apricots
- Walnuts
- Chia seeds
- Honey
- Shredded coconut (optional)

Instructions:
1. In a food processor, blend dried apricots, walnuts, chia seeds, and a drizzle of honey until a sticky mixture forms.
2. Roll into bite-sized balls.
3. Optionally, roll the balls in shredded coconut for added texture.
4. Refrigerate and enjoy these energy-packed bites.

---

24. Broccoli and Cheese Baked Potato

Ingredients:
- Baked sweet potato
- Steamed broccoli florets
- Shredded cheddar cheese
- Greek yogurt
- Chives, chopped

Instructions:
1. Cut open a baked sweet potato.
2. Top with steamed broccoli florets and shredded cheddar cheese.

3. Add a dollop of Greek yogurt and sprinkle with chopped chives.
4. Enjoy this nutrient-rich and calcium-loaded baked potato.

---

25. Peanut Butter and Banana Rice Cakes

Ingredients:
- Brown rice cakes
- Peanut butter
- Banana, sliced
- Chia seeds (optional)

Instructions:
1. Spread peanut butter over brown rice cakes.
2. Place banana slices on top.
3. Optionally, sprinkle with chia seeds for added crunch.
4. Savor this delicious and magnesium-rich snack.

---

26. Tomato Basil Bruschetta

Ingredients:
- Whole-grain baguette, sliced
- Fresh tomatoes, diced
- Fresh basil, chopped
- Olive oil
- Garlic, minced

Instructions:
1. Toast whole-grain baguette slices.
2. In a bowl, mix diced tomatoes, chopped basil, minced garlic, and a drizzle of olive oil.
3. Spoon the tomato mixture onto the toasted baguette slices.
4. Enjoy this flavorful and vitamin-rich bruschetta.

---

27. Celery Sticks with Almond Cream Cheese

Ingredients:
- Celery sticks
- Almond cream cheese
- Raisins

Instructions:
1. Fill celery sticks with almond cream cheese.
2. Top with raisins for a sweet and crunchy treat.
3. Savor this snack that combines calcium-rich ingredients with a hint of sweetness.

---

28. Minty Watermelon Salad

Ingredients:
- Watermelon, cubed
- Feta cheese, crumbled
- Fresh mint leaves, chopped
- Lime juice

Instructions:
1. Combine watermelon cubes, crumbled feta, and chopped fresh mint in a bowl.
2. Squeeze lime juice over the mixture.
3. Toss gently and enjoy this refreshing and calcium-packed watermelon salad.

---

29. Stuffed Dates with Almond Butter

Ingredients:
- Medjool dates, pitted
- Almond butter
- Walnuts, chopped

Instructions:
1. Open Medjool dates and remove pits.
2. Fill each date with a spoonful of almond butter.
3. Top with chopped walnuts for added crunch.
4. Savor these sweet and nutritious stuffed dates.

---

30. Spinach and Artichoke Dip with Whole-Grain Pita Chips

Ingredients:
- Fresh spinach, chopped
- Artichoke hearts, chopped
- Greek yogurt

- Parmesan cheese, grated
- Whole-grain pita bread, cut into triangles

Instructions:
1. In a bowl, mix chopped spinach, chopped artichoke hearts, Greek yogurt, and grated Parmesan cheese.
2. Bake until bubbly and golden.
3. Serve with whole-grain pita chips for a tasty and calcium-rich dip.

These detailed snack ideas provide a diverse range of flavors and nutrients for bone health. Enjoy these smart snacks as part of your Bone-Healthy Cooking journey!
 Chapter 5: Satisfying Sweets
-Certainly! Here are the first 10 satisfying and bone-healthy sweet treats for your cookbook:

---

 1. Chia Seed and Berry Pudding

Ingredients:
- Chia seeds
- Almond milk
- Mixed berries (strawberries, blueberries, raspberries)
- Maple syrup or honey

Instructions:
1. Mix chia seeds with almond milk and sweeten with maple syrup or honey.
2. Refrigerate until a pudding-like consistency forms.
3. Layer the chia pudding with mixed berries for a delightful and antioxidant-rich dessert.

---

2. Banana and Walnut Muffins

Ingredients:
- Ripe bananas, mashed
- Whole wheat flour
- Walnuts, chopped
- Greek yogurt
- Honey
- Baking powder

Instructions:
1. Combine mashed bananas, whole wheat flour, chopped walnuts, Greek yogurt, honey, and baking powder.
2. Spoon the batter into muffin cups and bake until golden.
3. Enjoy these wholesome banana and walnut muffins as a nutrient-packed dessert.

—

3. Yogurt Parfait with Granola and Berries

Ingredients:
- Greek yogurt
- Granola
- Mixed berries (blueberries, strawberries, raspberries)
- Honey

Instructions:
1. In a glass or bowl, layer Greek yogurt, granola, and mixed berries.
2. Drizzle with honey for added sweetness.
3. Savor this satisfying and calcium-rich yogurt parfait.

---

4. Dark Chocolate-Dipped Almonds

Ingredients:
- Dark chocolate, melted
- Almonds

Instructions:
1. Dip almonds into melted dark chocolate, ensuring they are fully coated.
2. Place on a parchment-lined tray and let the chocolate set.
3. Enjoy these crunchy and magnesium-rich dark chocolate-dipped almonds.

---

5. Baked Apples with Cinnamon and Walnuts

Ingredients:
- Apples, cored and sliced
- Cinnamon
- Walnuts, chopped
- Honey

Instructions:
1. Preheat the oven to 375°F (190°C).
2. Place apple slices in a baking dish and sprinkle with cinnamon.
3. Top with chopped walnuts and drizzle with honey.
4. Bake until apples are tender. Enjoy this warm and comforting dessert.

---

6. Coconut and Berry Smoothie Bowl

Ingredients:
- Coconut milk
- Mixed berries (strawberries, blueberries, raspberries)
- Shredded coconut
- Chia seeds

Instructions:
1. Blend coconut milk with mixed berries until smooth.
2. Pour the smoothie into a bowl and top with shredded coconut and chia seeds.
3. Enjoy this refreshing and nutrient-packed smoothie bowl.

---

7. Peach and Almond Crisp

Ingredients:
- Fresh peaches, sliced
- Almond flour
- Rolled oats
- Almonds, sliced
- Maple syrup

Instructions:
1. Arrange sliced peaches in a baking dish.
2. In a bowl, mix almond flour, rolled oats, sliced almonds, and maple syrup.
3. Spread the mixture over the peaches and bake until golden.
4. Serve this peach and almond crisp warm.

---

8. Frozen Yogurt Bites with Berries

Ingredients:
- Greek yogurt
- Mixed berries (blueberries, strawberries, raspberries)

Instructions:
1. Spoon Greek yogurt into bite-sized molds.
2. Press a few mixed berries into each mold.
3. Freeze until solid and enjoy these creamy and calcium-rich frozen yogurt bites.

---

9. Cocoa and Almond Energy Balls

Ingredients:
- Almonds
- Dates, pitted
- Cocoa powder
- Vanilla extract
- Shredded coconut (optional)

Instructions:
1. In a food processor, blend almonds, pitted dates, cocoa powder, and vanilla extract until a sticky mixture forms.
2. Roll into bite-sized balls.
3. Optionally, roll the balls in shredded coconut for added texture.
4. Refrigerate and enjoy these energy-packed cocoa and almond balls.

---

10. Mango Sorbet

Ingredients:
- Mango, diced
- Greek yogurt
- Honey
- Lime juice

Instructions:

1. Blend diced mango with Greek yogurt, honey, and lime juice until smooth.
2. Pour the mixture into a container and freeze until firm.
3. Scoop and enjoy this refreshing and vitamin C-rich mango sorbet.

These satisfying and bone-healthy sweet treats offer a mix of flavors while keeping nutritional value in mind. Enjoy these delicious desserts as part of your Bone-Healthy Cooking journey!Certainly! Here are the next 10 satisfying and bone-healthy sweet treats for your cookbook:

---

11. Blueberry and Almond Bliss Balls

Ingredients:
- Almonds
- Dried blueberries
- Chia seeds
- Honey

Instructions:
1. In a food processor, blend almonds, dried blueberries, chia seeds, and honey until a sticky mixture forms.
2. Roll into bite-sized bliss balls.
3. Refrigerate and enjoy these antioxidant-rich and energy-boosting treats.

---

12. Pumpkin Pie Smoothie

Ingredients:
- Pumpkin puree
- Almond milk
- Banana
- Cinnamon
- Nutmeg

Instructions:
1. Blend pumpkin puree, almond milk, banana, cinnamon, and nutmeg until smooth.
2. Pour into a glass and savor the flavors of a pumpkin pie in a healthy smoothie.

---

13. Almond and Apricot Oat Bars

Ingredients:
- Rolled oats
- Almond butter
- Dried apricots, chopped
- Maple syrup

Instructions:
1. Mix rolled oats, almond butter, chopped dried apricots, and maple syrup in a bowl.
2. Press the mixture into a baking dish and refrigerate until firm.

3. Cut into bars and enjoy these fiber-rich almond and apricot oat bars.

---

14. Cinnamon Baked Pears

Ingredients:
- Pears, halved and cored
- Cinnamon
- Walnuts, chopped
- Honey

Instructions:
1. Preheat the oven to 375°F (190°C).
2. Place pear halves in a baking dish, sprinkle with cinnamon, and top with chopped walnuts.
3. Drizzle with honey and bake until pears are tender.
4. Indulge in these warm and comforting cinnamon baked pears.

---

15. Raspberry and Yogurt Popsicles

Ingredients:
- Greek yogurt
- Fresh raspberries
- Honey

Instructions:

1. In a blender, mix Greek yogurt, fresh raspberries, and honey until smooth.
2. Pour the mixture into popsicle molds and freeze until solid.
3. Enjoy these refreshing and calcium-packed raspberry and yogurt popsicles.

---

16. Cranberry and Orange Granola Bars

Ingredients:
- Rolled oats
- Almonds, chopped
- Dried cranberries
- Orange zest
- Maple syrup

Instructions:
1. Combine rolled oats, chopped almonds, dried cranberries, orange zest, and maple syrup in a bowl.
2. Press the mixture into a baking dish and bake until golden.
3. Cut into bars and relish these tangy cranberry and orange granola bars.

---

17. Pistachio and Dark Chocolate Bark

Ingredients:
- Dark chocolate, melted
- Pistachios, chopped

- Dried cherries, chopped

Instructions:
1. Pour melted dark chocolate onto a parchment-lined tray.
2. Sprinkle chopped pistachios and dried cherries over the chocolate.
3. Let it set in the refrigerator, then break into pieces and enjoy this rich and antioxidant-filled bark.

---

18. Vanilla and Berry Chia Popsicles

Ingredients:
- Vanilla almond milk
- Mixed berries (strawberries, blueberries, raspberries)
- Chia seeds
- Maple syrup

Instructions:
1. Mix vanilla almond milk, mixed berries, chia seeds, and maple syrup in a blender.
2. Pour the mixture into popsicle molds and freeze until solid.
3. Delight in these creamy and chia-packed vanilla and berry popsicles.

---

19. Hazelnut and Fig Baked Apples

Ingredients:

- Apples, cored
- Hazelnuts, chopped
- Dried figs, chopped
- Cinnamon
- Honey

Instructions:
1. Preheat the oven to 375°F (190°C).
2. Mix chopped hazelnuts, dried figs, and a sprinkle of cinnamon.
3. Stuff cored apples with the mixture, drizzle with honey, and bake until apples are tender.
4. Enjoy these warm and nutty hazelnut and fig baked apples.

---

20. Mango and Coconut Rice Pudding

Ingredients:
- Arborio rice
- Coconut milk
- Mango, diced
- Agave syrup

Instructions:
1. Cook Arborio rice in coconut milk until creamy.
2. Stir in diced mango and sweeten with agave syrup.
3. Serve warm or chilled for a tropical and indulgent rice pudding.

Chapter 6: Beverage Bliss

1. Green Tea Infusion with Citrus Twist

Ingredients:
- Green tea bags
- Water
- Lemon slices
- Fresh mint leaves

Instructions:
1. Steep green tea bags in hot water.
2. Allow to cool, then refrigerate.
3. Serve over ice with lemon slices and fresh mint leaves for a revitalizing and antioxidant-rich beverage.

---

2. Berry Blast Smoothie

Ingredients:
- Mixed berries (strawberries, blueberries, raspberries)
- Greek yogurt
- Almond milk
- Chia seeds
- Honey

Instructions:
1. Blend mixed berries, Greek yogurt, almond milk, chia seeds, and honey until smooth.

2. Pour into a glass and enjoy this nutrient-packed and calcium-rich berry smoothie.

---

3. Turmeric Golden Milk Latte

Ingredients:
- Turmeric powder
- Almond milk
- Ginger, grated
- Cinnamon
- Honey

Instructions:
1. Mix turmeric powder, almond milk, grated ginger, and a sprinkle of cinnamon in a saucepan.
2. Heat until warm but not boiling.
3. Sweeten with honey for a soothing and anti-inflammatory turmeric golden milk latte.

---

4. Fresh Mint and Cucumber Infused Water

Ingredients:
- Fresh mint leaves
- Cucumber slices
- Water
- Ice cubes

Instructions:
1. Combine fresh mint leaves and cucumber slices in a pitcher.
2. Fill the pitcher with water and add ice cubes.
3. Let it infuse for a refreshing and hydrating mint and cucumber flavored water.

---

5. Citrus and Basil Sparkling Lemonade

Ingredients:
- Freshly squeezed lemon juice
- Orange slices
- Basil leaves
- Sparkling water
- Agave syrup

Instructions:
1. Mix freshly squeezed lemon juice, orange slices, and basil leaves in a pitcher.
2. Pour in sparkling water and sweeten with agave syrup to taste.
3. Enjoy this citrusy and herb-infused sparkling lemonade.

---

6. Pineapple and Ginger Tropical Smoothie

Ingredients:
- Pineapple chunks
- Coconut water
- Fresh ginger, grated

- Greek yogurt
- Flaxseeds

Instructions:
1. Blend pineapple chunks, coconut water, grated ginger, Greek yogurt, and flaxseeds until smooth.
2. Pour into a glass and savor this tropical and bone-healthy smoothie.

---

7. Hibiscus and Berry Iced Tea

Ingredients:
- Hibiscus tea bags
- Mixed berries (strawberries, blueberries, raspberries)
- Honey
- Ice cubes

Instructions:
1. Steep hibiscus tea bags in hot water, then let it cool.
2. Add mixed berries and honey to the tea.
3. Serve over ice for a refreshing and antioxidant-rich hibiscus and berry iced tea.

---

8. Watermelon and Mint Refresher

Ingredients:
- Fresh watermelon chunks

- Mint leaves
- Lime juice
- Coconut water

Instructions:
1. Blend fresh watermelon chunks, mint leaves, lime juice, and coconut water until smooth.
2. Strain if desired and serve over ice for a hydrating watermelon and mint refresher.

---

9. Cherry Almond Smoothie Bowl

Ingredients:
- Frozen cherries
- Almond milk
- Greek yogurt
- Almond butter
- Granola

Instructions:
1. Blend frozen cherries, almond milk, Greek yogurt, and almond butter until smooth.
2. Pour into a bowl and top with granola for a satisfying and calcium-rich smoothie bowl.

---

10. Matcha Green Tea Latte

Ingredients:
- Matcha powder
- Almond milk
- Honey
- Vanilla extract

Instructions:
1. Whisk matcha powder with a small amount of hot water until smooth.
2. Heat almond milk and whisk in the matcha mixture.
3. Sweeten with honey and add a splash of vanilla extract for a vibrant and antioxidant-packed matcha green tea latte.

---

11. Pomegranate and Blueberry Icy Elixir

Ingredients:
- Pomegranate juice
- Blueberries
- Ice cubes
- Fresh rosemary sprigs

Instructions:
1. Blend pomegranate juice and blueberries until smooth.
2. Strain the mixture and pour over ice.
3. Garnish with fresh rosemary sprigs for a cooling and antioxidant-rich elixir.

---

12. Coconut and Pineapple Smoothie

Ingredients:
- Coconut milk
- Pineapple chunks
- Banana
- Chia seeds
- Honey

Instructions:
1. Blend coconut milk, pineapple chunks, banana, chia seeds, and honey until creamy.
2. Pour into a glass and enjoy this tropical and bone-nourishing smoothie.

---

13. Minty Mango Limeade

Ingredients:
- Fresh mango, diced
- Lime juice
- Mint leaves
- Sparkling water
- Agave syrup

Instructions:
1. Muddle fresh mango, lime juice, and mint leaves in a glass.
2. Add sparkling water and sweeten with agave syrup.

3. Sip on this minty mango limeade for a refreshing and vitamin C-packed beverage.

---

14. Cherry and Basil Sparkling Water

Ingredients:
- Fresh cherries, pitted
- Basil leaves
- Sparkling water
- Lemon slices

Instructions:
1. Muddle fresh cherries and basil leaves in a glass.
2. Add sparkling water and garnish with lemon slices.
3. Enjoy this effervescent and antioxidant-rich cherry and basil sparkling water.

---

15. Cucumber and Melon Infused Detox Water

Ingredients:
- Cucumber slices
- Melon balls (cantaloupe, honeydew)
- Mint leaves
- Water
- Ice cubes

Instructions:

1. Combine cucumber slices, melon balls, and mint leaves in a pitcher.
2. Fill the pitcher with water and add ice cubes.
3. Let it infuse for a detoxifying and hydrating cucumber and melon flavored water.

---

16. Raspberry and Lemon Iced Green Tea

Ingredients:
- Green tea bags
- Water
- Fresh raspberries
- Lemon slices
- Honey

Instructions:
1. Steep green tea bags in hot water and let it cool.
2. Add fresh raspberries, lemon slices, and honey to the tea.
3. Serve over ice for a zesty and antioxidant-packed raspberry and lemon iced green tea.

---

17. Orange and Carrot Sunrise Smoothie

Ingredients:
- Oranges, peeled and segmented
- Carrots, chopped
- Greek yogurt

- Almond milk
- Turmeric powder

Instructions:
1. Blend oranges, carrots, Greek yogurt, almond milk, and turmeric powder until smooth.
2. Pour into a glass and enjoy this vibrant and vitamin-rich sunrise smoothie.

---

18. Peach and Raspberry Fizz

Ingredients:
- Fresh peaches, sliced
- Raspberries
- Sparkling water
- Fresh basil leaves

Instructions:
1. Muddle fresh peaches and raspberries in a glass.
2. Add sparkling water and garnish with fresh basil leaves.
3. Sip on this peach and raspberry fizz for a bubbly and fruity delight.

---

19. Blue Butterfly Pea Flower Tea

Ingredients:
- Blue butterfly pea flower tea bags

- Hot water
- Lemon wedges
- Honey

Instructions:
1. Steep blue butterfly pea flower tea bags in hot water.
2. Add lemon wedges and sweeten with honey.
3. Enjoy this visually stunning and antioxidant-rich blue tea.

---

20. Ginger-Lemon Elixir with Aloe Vera

Ingredients:
- Fresh ginger, grated
- Lemon juice
- Aloe vera gel
- Water
- Agave syrup

Instructions:
1. Mix grated fresh ginger, lemon juice, aloe vera gel, and water.
2. Sweeten with agave syrup to taste.
3. Sip on this invigorating ginger-lemon elixir with the added benefit of aloe vera.

-

Chapter 7: Calcium-Rich Creations

1. Spinach and Feta Stuffed Chicken Breast

Ingredients:
- Chicken breasts
- Fresh spinach
- Feta cheese, crumbled
- Garlic, minced
- Olive oil
- Lemon juice

Instructions:
1. Preheat the oven to 375°F (190°C).
2. Butterfly chicken breasts and stuff with a mixture of fresh spinach, crumbled feta, minced garlic, and a splash of olive oil.
3. Drizzle with lemon juice and bake until chicken is cooked through. Enjoy this protein-packed and calcium-rich creation.

---

2. Salmon and Broccoli Quinoa Bowl

Ingredients:
- Salmon fillets
- Quinoa
- Broccoli florets
- Lemon zest
- Olive oil
- Parmesan cheese, grated

Instructions:
1. Cook quinoa according to package instructions.
2. Grill or bake salmon fillets and steam broccoli florets.
3. Combine quinoa, salmon, and broccoli in a bowl. Drizzle with olive oil, sprinkle with lemon zest, and top with grated Parmesan. Indulge in this omega-3 and calcium-loaded quinoa bowl.

---

3. Cauliflower and Kale Gratin

Ingredients:
- Cauliflower, florets
- Kale, chopped
- Gruyere cheese, grated
- Milk
- Flour
- Butter

Instructions:
1. Steam cauliflower florets and sauté chopped kale until tender.
2. In a saucepan, make a cheese sauce by melting butter, adding flour, and then stirring in milk. Add grated Gruyere cheese until smooth.
3. Combine cauliflower, kale, and cheese sauce in a baking dish. Bake until golden. Savor this creamy and calcium-rich cauliflower and kale gratin.

---

4. Tofu and Broccoli Stir-Fry

Ingredients:
- Firm tofu, cubed
- Broccoli florets
- Soy sauce
- Garlic, minced
- Sesame oil
- Brown rice

Instructions:
1. Sauté cubed tofu in sesame oil until golden. Add minced garlic.
2. Steam broccoli until crisp-tender.
3. Combine tofu and broccoli in a stir-fry with soy sauce. Serve over brown rice for a plant-based and calcium-packed creation.

---

5. Mushroom and Swiss Chard Omelette

Ingredients:
- Eggs
- Mushrooms, sliced
- Swiss chard, chopped
- Swiss cheese, grated
- Olive oil
- Salt and pepper

Instructions:
1. Sauté sliced mushrooms and chopped Swiss chard in olive oil until tender.

2. Beat eggs and pour over the vegetables. Sprinkle with grated Swiss cheese.
3. Cook until the eggs are set. Fold and enjoy this protein and calcium-rich mushroom and Swiss chard omelette.

---

6. Greek Yogurt Parfait with Berries and Almonds

Ingredients:
- Greek yogurt
- Mixed berries (blueberries, strawberries, raspberries)
- Almonds, sliced
- Honey

Instructions:
1. Layer Greek yogurt with mixed berries and sliced almonds in a glass.
2. Drizzle with honey for a delicious and calcium-loaded parfait.

---

7. Cheesy Spinach and Artichoke Dip

Ingredients:
- Fresh spinach, chopped
- Artichoke hearts, chopped
- Cream cheese
- Sour cream
- Parmesan cheese, grated
- Garlic, minced

Instructions:
1. Mix chopped spinach, chopped artichoke hearts, cream cheese, sour cream, grated Parmesan, and minced garlic.
2. Bake until bubbly and serve with whole-grain pita chips. Relish in this creamy and calcium-rich spinach and artichoke dip.

---

8. Cottage Cheese and Fruit Salad

Ingredients:
- Cottage cheese
- Fresh fruit (pineapple, mango, kiwi)
- Mint leaves, chopped
- Almond slices

Instructions:
1. Combine cottage cheese with fresh fruit chunks in a bowl.
2. Sprinkle with chopped mint leaves and almond slices for a refreshing and calcium-rich fruit salad.

---

9. Shrimp and Asparagus Risotto

Ingredients:
- Arborio rice
- Shrimp, peeled and deveined
- Asparagus, chopped
- Chicken broth

- White wine
- Parmesan cheese, grated

Instructions:
1. Sauté shrimp and asparagus in a pan until shrimp are pink and asparagus is tender.
2. Cook Arborio rice in chicken broth and white wine until creamy.
3. Stir in the shrimp, asparagus, and grated Parmesan. Enjoy this delectable and calcium-packed shrimp and asparagus risotto.

---

10. Avocado and Kale Smoothie Bowl

Ingredients:
- Kale leaves, stems removed
- Avocado
- Banana
- Almond milk
- Chia seeds

Instructions:
1. Blend kale leaves, avocado, banana, and almond milk until smooth.
2. Pour into a bowl and top with chia seeds for a nutrient-rich and calcium-loaded smoothie bowl.

---

11. Salmon and Spinach Stuffed Portobello Mushrooms

Ingredients:
- Portobello mushrooms
- Salmon fillet, cooked and flaked
- Fresh spinach, sautéed
- Feta cheese, crumbled
- Olive oil
- Lemon zest

Instructions:
1. Remove the stems from portobello mushrooms and brush with olive oil.
2. Fill mushrooms with a mixture of cooked and flaked salmon, sautéed spinach, and crumbled feta.
3. Bake until mushrooms are tender. Garnish with lemon zest and enjoy this savory and calcium-rich creation.

---

12. Quinoa and Kale Stuffed Bell Peppers

Ingredients:
- Bell peppers, halved
- Quinoa, cooked
- Kale, chopped and sautéed
- Black beans, drained and rinsed
- Cheddar cheese, shredded
- Tomato salsa

Instructions:
1. Preheat the oven to 375°F (190°C).
2. Fill halved bell peppers with a mixture of cooked quinoa, sautéed kale, black beans, and shredded cheddar cheese.
3. Bake until peppers are tender. Serve with tomato salsa for a protein and calcium-packed dish.

---

13. Broccoli and Cheese Stuffed Baked Potatoes

Ingredients:
- Russet potatoes, baked
- Broccoli florets, steamed
- Cheddar cheese, shredded
- Greek yogurt
- Chives, chopped
- Salt and pepper

Instructions:
1. Scoop out the flesh of baked potatoes and mash with steamed broccoli, shredded cheddar cheese, Greek yogurt, chives, salt, and pepper.
2. Refill the potato skins and bake until cheese is melted. Relish in these cheesy and calcium-rich stuffed baked potatoes.

---

14. Pumpkin Seed and Spinach Pesto Pasta

Ingredients:
- Whole wheat pasta
- Pumpkin seeds, toasted
- Fresh spinach
- Parmesan cheese, grated
- Garlic
- Olive oil

Instructions:
1. Cook whole wheat pasta according to package instructions.
2. In a food processor, blend toasted pumpkin seeds, fresh spinach, grated Parmesan, garlic, and olive oil into a pesto.
3. Toss the pesto with the cooked pasta for a nutty and calcium-packed dish.

---

15. Chicken and Broccoli Alfredo

Ingredients:
- Fettuccine pasta
- Chicken breasts, grilled and sliced
- Broccoli florets, steamed
- Alfredo sauce
- Parmesan cheese, grated
- Black pepper

Instructions:
1. Cook fettuccine pasta according to package instructions.

2. Mix grilled and sliced chicken, steamed broccoli, Alfredo sauce, and grated Parmesan in a pan.
3. Combine with cooked pasta and sprinkle with black pepper. Enjoy this creamy and calcium-rich chicken and broccoli Alfredo.

---

16. Sesame-Crusted Tofu with Bok Choy

Ingredients:
- Firm tofu, sliced
- Sesame seeds
- Bok choy, sautéed
- Soy sauce
- Ginger, grated
- Sesame oil

Instructions:
1. Coat tofu slices with sesame seeds and pan-sear until golden.
2. Sauté bok choy with soy sauce, grated ginger, and a splash of sesame oil.
3. Serve sesame-crusted tofu over sautéed bok choy for a plant-based and calcium-packed delight.

---

17. Brussels Sprouts and Walnut Salad

Ingredients:
- Brussels sprouts, shaved
- Walnuts, toasted

- Pomegranate seeds
- Feta cheese, crumbled
- Balsamic vinaigrette
- Dijon mustard

Instructions:
1. Shave Brussels sprouts and toss with toasted walnuts, pomegranate seeds, and crumbled feta.
2. Whisk together balsamic vinaigrette and Dijon mustard, then drizzle over the salad. Enjoy this crunchy and calcium-rich Brussels sprouts and walnut salad.

---

18. Chickpea and Spinach Curry

Ingredients:
- Chickpeas, cooked
- Fresh spinach
- Tomatoes, diced
- Coconut milk
- Curry powder
- Garlic, minced

Instructions:
1. Sauté minced garlic in a pan, add cooked chickpeas, diced tomatoes, fresh spinach, and coconut milk.
2. Stir in curry powder and simmer until the spinach wilts. Serve over rice for a flavorful and calcium-rich chickpea and spinach curry.

---

19. Eggplant Parmesan

Ingredients:
- Eggplant, sliced
- Marinara sauce
- Mozzarella cheese, shredded
- Parmesan cheese, grated
- Fresh basil leaves
- Olive oil

Instructions:
1. Coat eggplant slices in olive oil and bake until golden.
2. Layer baked eggplant with marinara sauce, shredded mozzarella, and grated Parmesan.
3. Bake until cheese is melted and bubbly. Garnish with fresh basil for a cheesy and calcium-loaded eggplant Parmesan.

---

20. Artichoke and Ricotta Stuffed Shells

Ingredients:
- Jumbo pasta shells, cooked
- Artichoke hearts, chopped
- Ricotta cheese
- Spinach, chopped
- Marinara sauce
- Pecorino Romano cheese, grated

Instructions:
1. Combine chopped artichoke hearts, ricotta cheese, and chopped spinach.
2. Stuff cooked pasta shells with the mixture and place in a baking dish.
3. Pour marinara sauce over the shells, sprinkle with grated Pecorino Romano, and bake until bubbly. Savor these delicious and calcium-rich artichoke and ricotta stuffed shells.

Chapter 8: Vitamin D Delights

1. Sunshine Smoothie Bowl

Ingredients:
- Greek yogurt
- Mango chunks
- Pineapple slices
- Chia seeds
- Almond milk
- Granola

Instructions:
1. Blend Greek yogurt, mango chunks, pineapple slices, chia seeds, and almond milk until smooth.
2. Pour into a bowl and top with granola for a tropical and Vitamin D-packed smoothie bowl.

---

2. Smoked Salmon and Avocado Toast

Ingredients:
- Whole-grain bread
- Smoked salmon
- Avocado slices
- Cream cheese
- Dill
- Lemon zest

Instructions:
1. Toast whole-grain bread and spread cream cheese.
2. Top with smoked salmon, avocado slices, dill, and a sprinkle of lemon zest. Enjoy this savory and Vitamin D-rich toast.

---

3. Vitamin D Boosting Omelette

Ingredients:
- Eggs
- Shiitake mushrooms, sliced
- Spinach leaves
- Feta cheese, crumbled
- Olive oil
- Salt and pepper

Instructions:
1. Sauté sliced shiitake mushrooms in olive oil until golden.
2. Beat eggs and pour over the mushrooms. Add spinach leaves and crumbled feta.
3. Cook until the eggs are set. Fold and relish this protein and Vitamin D-packed omelette.

---

4. Sardine and Tomato Bruschetta

Ingredients:
- Sardines in olive oil
- Cherry tomatoes, halved

- Whole-grain baguette slices
- Basil leaves
- Balsamic glaze

Instructions:
1. Toast whole-grain baguette slices and top with sardines, halved cherry tomatoes, and basil leaves.
2. Drizzle with balsamic glaze for a Mediterranean-inspired and Vitamin D-rich bruschetta.

---

5. Grilled Portobello Mushrooms with Egg

Ingredients:
- Portobello mushrooms
- Eggs
- Cherry tomatoes, sliced
- Parmesan cheese, grated
- Olive oil
- Fresh thyme

Instructions:
1. Grill portobello mushrooms and crack an egg into each cap.
2. Top with sliced cherry tomatoes, grated Parmesan, and a drizzle of olive oil.
3. Grill until the eggs are cooked. Sprinkle with fresh thyme and savor these grilled and Vitamin D-rich portobello mushrooms.

---

6. Vitamin D Citrus Salad

Ingredients:
- Spinach leaves
- Orange segments
- Grapefruit segments
- Avocado slices
- Walnuts, toasted
- Citrus vinaigrette

Instructions:
1. Toss spinach leaves with orange and grapefruit segments, avocado slices, and toasted walnuts.
2. Drizzle with citrus vinaigrette for a refreshing and Vitamin D-packed citrus salad.

---

7. Mushroom and Cheese Stuffed Mini Peppers

Ingredients:
- Mini bell peppers, halved
- Cremini mushrooms, chopped
- Mozzarella cheese, shredded
- Garlic, minced
- Olive oil
- Fresh parsley

Instructions:
1. Sauté chopped cremini mushrooms with minced garlic in olive oil until tender.

2. Stuff mini bell peppers with the mushroom mixture and top with shredded mozzarella.
3. Bake until cheese is melted and bubbly. Garnish with fresh parsley for a delightful and Vitamin D-rich appetizer.

---

8. Salmon and Dill Pasta Salad

Ingredients:
- Whole-grain pasta
- Canned salmon, flaked
- Cherry tomatoes, halved
- Cucumber, diced
- Fresh dill, chopped
- Greek yogurt dressing

Instructions:
1. Cook whole-grain pasta and toss with flaked canned salmon, cherry tomatoes, diced cucumber, and chopped fresh dill.
2. Drizzle with a Greek yogurt dressing for a satisfying and Vitamin D-rich pasta salad.

---

9. Shrimp and Mango Summer Rolls

Ingredients:
- Rice paper wrappers
- Shrimp, cooked and peeled
- Mango, julienned

- Avocado slices
- Fresh mint leaves
- Peanut dipping sauce

Instructions:
1. Soak rice paper wrappers in warm water until pliable.
2. Fill each wrapper with cooked shrimp, julienned mango, avocado slices, and fresh mint leaves.
3. Roll tightly and serve with peanut dipping sauce for a light and Vitamin D-packed summer roll.

---

10. Canned Tuna and Quinoa Bowl

Ingredients:
- Quinoa, cooked
- Canned tuna, drained
- Cherry tomatoes, halved
- Kalamata olives, sliced
- Feta cheese, crumbled
- Lemon vinaigrette

Instructions:
1. Mix cooked quinoa with drained canned tuna, halved cherry tomatoes, sliced Kalamata olives, and crumbled feta.
2. Drizzle with lemon vinaigrette for a quick and Vitamin D-rich quinoa bowl.

---

11. Grilled Swordfish with Lemon-Herb Marinade

Ingredients:
- Swordfish steaks
- Lemon juice
- Olive oil
- Fresh herbs (such as thyme, rosemary, and parsley)
- Garlic, minced
- Salt and pepper

Instructions:
1. Marinate swordfish steaks in a mixture of lemon juice, olive oil, minced garlic, fresh herbs, salt, and pepper.
2. Grill until the fish is cooked through. Serve with a squeeze of lemon for a flavorful and Vitamin D-rich dish.

---

12. Vitamin D-Infused Avocado Toast

Ingredients:
- Whole-grain bread
- Avocado
- Poached egg
- Chili flakes
- Lemon zest
- Salt and pepper

Instructions:
1. Toast whole-grain bread and spread ripe avocado.

2. Top with a poached egg, sprinkle with chili flakes, lemon zest, salt, and pepper. Enjoy this tasty and Vitamin D-infused avocado toast.

---

13. Baked Cod with Tomato and Olive Relish

Ingredients:
- Cod fillets
- Cherry tomatoes, halved
- Kalamata olives, sliced
- Red onion, finely chopped
- Fresh basil, chopped
- Balsamic glaze

Instructions:
1. Place cod fillets on a baking sheet.
2. Mix cherry tomatoes, Kalamata olives, red onion, and fresh basil. Spoon over the cod.
3. Bake until the fish is flaky. Drizzle with balsamic glaze for a Mediterranean-inspired and Vitamin D-rich baked cod.

---

14. Sun-Dried Tomato and Feta Stuffed Chicken Breast

Ingredients:
- Chicken breasts
- Sun-dried tomatoes, chopped
- Feta cheese, crumbled

- Spinach leaves
- Olive oil
- Italian seasoning

Instructions:
1. Preheat the oven to 375°F (190°C).
2. Cut a pocket in each chicken breast and stuff with sun-dried tomatoes, feta cheese, and spinach.
3. Drizzle with olive oil, sprinkle with Italian seasoning, and bake until the chicken is cooked through. Savor this savory and Vitamin D-rich stuffed chicken breast.

---

15. Mushroom and Swiss Chard Frittata

Ingredients:
- Eggs
- Mushrooms, sliced
- Swiss chard, chopped
- Swiss cheese, grated
- Onion, diced
- Olive oil

Instructions:
1. Sauté sliced mushrooms, chopped Swiss chard, and diced onion in olive oil until tender.
2. Beat eggs and pour over the vegetables. Top with grated Swiss cheese.
3. Cook until the eggs are set. Slice and enjoy this flavorful and Vitamin D-packed frittata.

---

16. Caprese Salad with Grilled Tofu

Ingredients:
- Tofu, sliced and grilled
- Cherry tomatoes, halved
- Fresh mozzarella, sliced
- Basil leaves
- Balsamic glaze
- Olive oil

Instructions:
1. Grill tofu slices until golden.
2. Arrange grilled tofu, cherry tomatoes, fresh mozzarella, and basil leaves on a plate.
3. Drizzle with balsamic glaze and olive oil for a light and Vitamin D-rich Caprese salad.

---

17. Creamy Salmon and Spinach Pasta

Ingredients:
- Whole-grain pasta
- Salmon fillet, cooked and flaked
- Fresh spinach leaves
- Cream cheese
- Lemon zest
- Dill

Instructions:
1. Cook whole-grain pasta and toss with cooked and flaked salmon and fresh spinach leaves.
2. Stir in cream cheese, lemon zest, and dill until creamy. Enjoy this creamy and Vitamin D-infused salmon and spinach pasta.

---

18. Vitamin D Boosting Tuna Salad Wraps

Ingredients:
- Canned tuna, drained
- Greek yogurt
- Cucumber, diced
- Red bell pepper, diced
- Whole-grain wraps
- Lettuce leaves

Instructions:
1. Mix drained canned tuna with Greek yogurt, diced cucumber, and diced red bell pepper.
2. Spoon the tuna mixture onto whole-grain wraps, add lettuce leaves, and wrap into a delicious and Vitamin D-boosting tuna salad.

---

19. Sesame-Crusted Salmon with Orange Glaze

Ingredients:
- Salmon fillets

- Sesame seeds
- Orange juice
- Soy sauce
- Honey
- Garlic, minced

Instructions:
1. Coat salmon fillets with sesame seeds and sear until golden.
2. Mix orange juice, soy sauce, honey, and minced garlic into a glaze.
3. Drizzle the glaze over the sesame-crusted salmon for a sweet and Vitamin D-rich dish.

---

20. Mango-Coconut Chia Pudding

Ingredients:
- Chia seeds
- Coconut milk
- Mango, diced
- Shredded coconut
- Agave syrup

Instructions:
1. Mix chia seeds with coconut milk and let it sit until it thickens.
2. Layer chia pudding with diced mango in a glass.
3. Sprinkle with shredded coconut and drizzle with agave syrup for a tropical and Vitamin D-infused chia pudding.

Chapter 9: Magnesium and Phosphorus Marvels

1. Quinoa and Black Bean Stuffed Bell Peppers

Ingredients:
- Bell peppers, halved
- Quinoa, cooked
- Black beans, cooked and drained
- Corn kernels
- Avocado, diced
- Cilantro, chopped

Instructions:
1. Preheat the oven to 375°F (190°C).
2. Mix cooked quinoa, black beans, corn, diced avocado, and chopped cilantro.
3. Stuff bell peppers with the mixture and bake until peppers are tender. Enjoy this protein-packed and magnesium-rich stuffed bell pepper.

---

2. Salmon and Asparagus Foil Packets

Ingredients:
- Salmon fillets
- Asparagus spears
- Lemon slices
- Garlic, minced
- Olive oil

- Dill

Instructions:
1. Preheat the oven to 400°F (200°C).
2. Place salmon fillets on foil, add asparagus, lemon slices, minced garlic, olive oil, and dill.
3. Seal the foil packets and bake until the salmon is cooked through. Savor this flavorful and phosphorus-rich salmon and asparagus dish.

---

3. Brown Rice and Lentil Buddha Bowl

Ingredients:
- Brown rice, cooked
- Lentils, cooked
- Spinach leaves
- Cherry tomatoes, halved
- Feta cheese, crumbled
- Tahini dressing

Instructions:
1. Arrange cooked brown rice, lentils, spinach leaves, halved cherry tomatoes, and crumbled feta in a bowl.
2. Drizzle with tahini dressing for a nourishing and magnesium-packed Buddha bowl.

—

4. Almond-Crusted Chicken Tenders

Ingredients:
- Chicken tenders
- Almonds, ground
- Egg
- Whole wheat flour
- Garlic powder
- Paprika

Instructions:
1. Preheat the oven to 400°F (200°C).
2. Dip chicken tenders in whisked egg, coat with a mixture of ground almonds, whole wheat flour, garlic powder, and paprika.
3. Bake until chicken is cooked and enjoy these crunchy and magnesium-rich almond-crusted chicken tenders.

---

5. Greek Yogurt and Berry Parfait

Ingredients:
- Greek yogurt
- Mixed berries (blueberries, strawberries, raspberries)
- Granola
- Chia seeds
- Honey

Instructions:
1. Layer Greek yogurt with mixed berries, granola, chia seeds, and a drizzle of honey for a delicious and phosphorus-rich parfait.

---

6. Mango and Avocado Spinach Salad

Ingredients:
- Spinach leaves
- Mango, diced
- Avocado, sliced
- Pomegranate seeds
- Walnuts, chopped
- Balsamic vinaigrette

Instructions:
1. Toss spinach leaves with diced mango, sliced avocado, pomegranate seeds, and chopped walnuts.
2. Drizzle with balsamic vinaigrette for a refreshing and magnesium-packed spinach salad.

---

7. Crispy Baked Sweet Potato Wedges

Ingredients:
- Sweet potatoes, cut into wedges
- Olive oil
- Smoked paprika
- Garlic powder
- Sea salt

Instructions:
1. Preheat the oven to 425°F (220°C).

2. Toss sweet potato wedges with olive oil, smoked paprika, garlic powder, and sea salt.
3. Bake until crispy and enjoy these delicious and phosphorus-rich sweet potato wedges.

---

8. Chia Seed and Almond Milk Pudding

Ingredients:
- Chia seeds
- Almond milk
- Vanilla extract
- Maple syrup
- Sliced almonds
- Fresh berries

Instructions:
1. Mix chia seeds with almond milk, vanilla extract, and maple syrup. Let it refrigerate until it thickens.
2. Top with sliced almonds and fresh berries for a nutritious and magnesium-packed chia seed pudding.

---

9. Broccoli and Chickpea Stir-Fry

Ingredients:
- Broccoli florets
- Chickpeas, cooked
- Red bell pepper, sliced

- Soy sauce
- Sesame oil
- Ginger, grated

Instructions:
1. Sauté broccoli florets, cooked chickpeas, and sliced red bell pepper in sesame oil with grated ginger.
2. Add soy sauce and stir-fry until the vegetables are tender. Enjoy this quick and magnesium-rich broccoli and chickpea stir-fry.

---

10. Tahini and Pumpkin Seed Hummus

Ingredients:
- Chickpeas, drained and rinsed
- Tahini
- Pumpkin seeds
- Lemon juice
- Garlic, minced
- Olive oil

Instructions:
1. Blend chickpeas, tahini, pumpkin seeds, lemon juice, minced garlic, and olive oil until smooth.
2. Serve as a dip with vegetable sticks or whole-grain crackers for a delicious and phosphorus-packed snack.

Conclusion

In concluding this culinary journey through the pages of the "Osteoporosis Diet Cookbook for Seniors Over 60," we have woven a tapestry of flavors, nutrition, and the shared joy of good food. This cookbook stands as a testament to the belief that eating well is not just a necessity but a celebration, especially as we gracefully navigate the golden years.

In each chapter, from sunrise breakfasts to comforting dinners and the delightful in-between, we've strived to create recipes that resonate with the unique tastes and nutritional needs of our seniors. The kitchen, often considered the heart of a home, becomes the canvas where we paint vibrant portraits of health, vitality, and the pure pleasure derived from nourishing the body and the spirit.

Within these pages, we've explored the nuances of osteoporosis, unwrapped the significance of essential nutrients, and offered a guide to crafting meals that contribute to bone health. It's not just a cookbook; it's a companion on the journey to embracing wellness, longevity, and the sheer joy found in relishing a meal made with care.

As you turn the last page, may this cookbook continue to inspire culinary adventures, encourage shared moments around the table, and, above all, foster a commitment to the well-being of our beloved seniors. Here's to savoring the richness of life, one delectable recipe at a time.

Cheers!!!